Experimentelle Medizin, Pathologie und Klinik

Band 25

Herausgegeben von

R. Hegglin · F. Leuthardt · R. Schoen · H. Schwiegk
A. Studer · H. U. Zollinger

Max W. Hess

Experimental Thymectomy
Possibilities and Limitations

With 7 Figures

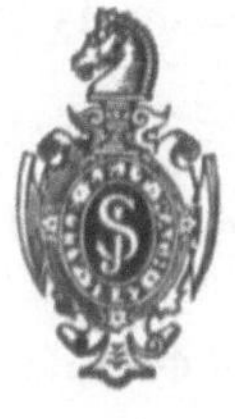

Springer-Verlag Berlin · Heidelberg · New York 1968

Max Walter Hess, M.D.
Theodor Kocher Institute, Institute of Pathology, University of Bern and
Medical Research Center, Brookhaven National Laboratory, Upton, N.Y.

ISBN-13: 978-3-642-86676-0   e-ISBN-13: 978-3-642-86675-3
DOI: 10.1007/ 978-3-642-86675-3

Library of Congress Catalog Card Number 68-31624

The use of general descriptive names, trade names, trade marks, etc. in this publication, even if the
former are not especially identified, is not to be taken as a sign that such names, as understood by
the Trade Marks and Merchandise Marks Act, may accordingly be used freely by anyone

Title-No. 6548

Foreword

Since the interest on the thymus as an organ essential for the development of immunological capacity was renewed more than ten years ago, the search for a better understanding of the mechanisms underlying its functions has not come to an end. Although the first observations suggesting a link between the thymus and immunocompetence related to certain clinical disorders in man such as thymoma or Swiss type of agammaglobulinemia, the bulk of evidence demonstrating the role of this lymphoepithelial organ in immune reactivity originates from experimental work as initiated by Dr. MILLER and Dr. GOOD's group. The full significance of the thymic system is now beginning to unfold. The basic question to be answered by the many investigators in the field is no longer whether the thymus does in fact play the role of an immunologically important organ but rather how it acts. In addition we need to know in what period(s) of ontogenesis is a proper development of the thymus a prerequisit for the buildup of an efficient peripheral lymphoreticular system throughout the organism.

Perinatal thymectomy proved to be a valuable experimental approach to gain a better insight into thymic functions. At first it looked as if this measure, in most of the species tested, would largely depress or abolish all immune reactions of the animal and lead to an inescapable wasting syndrome within a few months. It became apparent, however, that the latter phenomenon is due mainly to infection since wasting was not observed in animals kept under specific pathogen-free or germfree conditions, and could, at least in part, be reversed by antibiotic treatment. Characteristically, perinatally thymectomized specific pathogen free or germfree animals exhibit only a moderate depression of their capacity to react to strong antigenic challenges; this seems to be true for both their ability to produce humoral antibody, at least against certain antigens, and their capability to reject homografts. It now appears as an attractive hypothesis that perinatal thymectomy in most species is not followed by complete abolition of the immune capacities because it occurs too late in ontogenesis. The defects observed in Swiss type of agammaglobulinemia in man have so far not been simulated by animal experiments.

The work of Drs. HESS and STONER has contributed significantly to the present understanding of thymic functions in mammals, both in respect to antibody formation and also with regard to the importance of thymic cell emigration. Although many problems such as the possible role of the thymus in endowing undifferentiated lymphoid cells ("stem cells") with immunocompetence, or the elaboration of humoral factors by thymic epithelial cells, remain to be clarified, it seemed important to reevaluate the present state of knowledge in the field. It will be noted that several of the author's views differ to some extent from opinions expressed earlier by other workers: such a dialogue, confronting facts and contrasting working hypotheses, has always been refreshing and helpful in advancing our understanding of biological processes. The present monograph is an excellent example of a careful examination and critical consideration of relevant findings in thymus research, a considerable number of which have been made by the author himself. In particular, Dr. HESS may be congratulated for having stated so clearly what may be considered as established facts and what questions remain to be answered. Such is a good basis for choosing future research lines to follow.

Bern, May 1968   H. COTTIER, M. D.

Acknowledgments

The author is indebted to Prof. H. COTTIER and Dr. R. D. STONER for invaluable help and criticism.

Most of the experimental work was carried out at the Medical Research Center, Brookhaven National Laboratory, Upton, L. I., N. Y., under support by the U.S. Atomic Energy Commission.

During completion of the manuscript the author was financially supported by grants from the Swiss National Foundation for Scientific Research.

Springer Publishers should be commended for most pleasant cooperation and efficient publication.

M. W. HESS

Contents

1. Introduction

The thymus has long been considered an enigmatic organ. During the past
10 years of active research on the thymus a host of functions has been
ascribed to it; for reviews of older literature with its many contradictory
reports see MATTI (1911), PAPPENHEIMER (1914 a), PARK and McCLURE
(1919), ANDERSEN (1932), HAMMAR (1936), TESSERAUX (1953), ARNASON
et al. (1962) and MILLER and DUKOR (1964).

Based on the observation that the organ is large in newborn and young
animals while it is involuted and barely discernible in adult animals, an
intimate involvement of the thymus in growth regulation was assumed. Inhibition of body growth, sometimes associated with ossification defects,
osteoporosis or hypoplasia of developing bones, was observed in thymectomized animals; both stimulation and/or inhibition of growth was reported in animals fed thymic extracts or carrying thymus implants (KLOSE
and VOGT, 1910; TESSERAUX, 1953). The controversial concept of growth
regulation by the thymus has been devaluated by studies indicating that the
reported defects were accidental: thymectomized animals were found to be
very susceptible to infection (KLOSE and VOGT, 1910; HELLMAN and WHITE,
1930; COMSA, 1957), and the defects in bone development and structure
were probably due to ablation of the parathyroid (PAPPENHEIMER, 1914 b).
SZENT-GYORGYI et al. (1963) recently described the isolation of both a
growth-promoting ("promine") and growth-inhibiting substance ("retine")
from thymic tissue. These substances appear not to be thymus-specific, however, since they could be isolated from muscle tissue, tendons and arterial
walls as well.

The thymus was also believed to produce a substance influencing sexual
maturation; metamorphosis of amphibians was delayed or completely inhibited when the larvae were fed thymic extracts, puberty could occasion-
ally be precipitated by thymectomy in young mammals, and castrates were
shown to retain large thymic organs throughout adulthood. In addition, a
synergistic and an antagonistic action of the thymus on other endocrine
systems were reported (adrenals, thyroid, parathyroid, pancreas, hypophysis, pineal gland). The mutual interaction between the thymus and
various endocrine organs appears to be very complex. In suitably controlled
studies no effect of thymectomy was observed on sexual maturation or function (ANDERSEN, 1932). Testosterone and estrogens cause the thymus to in-

volute (MARINE et al., 1924; KAPLAN, 1954). Thymus hyperplasia following adrenalectomy and in Addison's disease has been described (PAPPENHEIMER, 1914 a); corticosteroids cause an acute thymic involution (DOUGHERTY, 1952). More recently, acute thymic involution was also described to occur following hypophysectomy in mice (PIERPAOLI and SORKIN, 1967). The essence of these studies indicates no more than that the thymus may respond to various hormonal influences or changes produced by them; through these mechanisms some degree of control may be exerted over the cellular make-up of the lymphoid tissue as a whole, and over the thymus in particular.

Pediatricians created the concept of "status thymico-lymphaticus" in which thymic and lymphoid hyperplasia were held responsible for unexplained sudden deaths in small children. Monographs have been written on the subject (HART, 1923; THOMAS, 1927), and "status thymico-lymphaticus" was discussed at various congresses (see HAMMAR, 1930; MITCHELL et al., 1939). HAMMAR (1929) and ROESSLE and ROULET (1931) established that reference values for thymic weights in children were, as a rule, too low since they were based on weight measurements on involuted thymic tissue from autopsied children which had died from infection or from other consumptive diseases. According to the reference weights of HAMMAR and ROESSLE and ROULET, children dying from so-called "status thymico-lymphaticus" had no thymic hyperplasia. Nevertheless, this misconception apparently is difficult to eradicate, and the diagnosis of thymic death is still being used at present. According to POTTER (1948) this "hoax" will disappear only if and when someone detects the specific function of the thymus.

A more fruitful approach towards elucidation of the enigmatic function(s) of the thymus was initiated with the concept that the thymus may be an important site for production of lymphocytes (BEARD, 1895; AUERBACH, 1960). A fall in the peripheral blood lymphocytes was observed following thymectomy in rats (PATON and GOODALL, 1904; SANDERS and FLOREY, 1940; REINHARDT, 1945; SCHOOLEY and KELLY, 1961), mice (METCALF, 1960; MILLER, 1961), guinea pigs (PATON and GOODALL, 1904; COMSA, 1957; REINHARDT and YOFFEY, 1956), rabbits (SANDERS and FLOREY, 1940; NAKAMOTO, 1957 a), dogs (KLOSE, 1914), and man (JOSKE, 1958). HAMMAR (1938) postulated involvement of the thymus in immune reactions. He thought that vitamin C was influencing immune reactivity and that it was produced in great quantities in Hassall's bodies; at the time of puberty, the decreasing production of vitamin C by the involuting thymus would be balanced by similarly beneficial effects on immune processes of sex hormones. Although he was unable to demonstrate a statistically significant depression in the ability of adult thymectomized rabbits to form antibodies against *Salmonella* antigen, he advanced the idea that the function of the thymus might be better understood if thymectomy was performed earlier in the life of the animals.

HAMMAR'S idea was forgotten for more than 20 years until a series of
incidental observations made in different laboratories set the stage for the
enormously increased activity in thymus research which could be witnessed
during the last years. The first of these observations was reported by GOOD
and VARCO (1955): a patient with a benign thymoma had developed a
marked immunologic deficiency, and was found to have extremely low
levels of gamma globulin in his serum; removal of the epithelial tumor
failed to alter the hypogammaglobulinemic state or the immunologic defect.
Subsequent to the report of GOOD and VARCO a series of other cases with a
combination of thymoma and agammaglobulinemia were observed (see
BARANDUN et al., 1959; JEUNET, 1965; GABRIELSEN and GOOD, 1966; GOOD
et al., 1967). COTTIER (1957) suggested that both morphological and immunological deficiency in patients with Swiss type agammaglobulinemia were
related to a developmental defect of the thymus, since in these cases the
thymus is extremely small, poorly developed and does not complete its
descensus. At about that time, a chance observation by GLICK and associates
(CHANG et al., 1955; GLICK et al., 1956) linked the bursa of Fabricius to
the development of antibody-forming capacity in newly hatched chickens.
Since the bursa of the birds closely resembles the thymus, MUELLER et al.
(1960) suggested that neonatal thymectomy in mammals might have similar
effects on immune reactivity as bursectomy in newly-hatched birds. Three
independent reports on results obtained in neonatally thymectomized animals followed each other very shortly. ARCHER and PIERCE (1961) observed
inability of neonatally thymectomized rabbits to produce antibodies against
bovine serum albumin; MILLER (1961) who was originally working on
problems of murine leukemia thymectomized newborn mice and found them
to be unable to reject skin homografts; and FICHTELIUS et al. (1961) found
an impairment of primary responses following stimulation with *Salmonella
typhi* in young adult guinea pigs which had been partially thymectomized.

During more recent years many publications appeared in which the
possible function(s) of the thymus were analyzed experimentally or solely
in a speculative manner. The abundance of highly diversified information
gained through these studies is confusing and has been the subject of various
reviews and conferences (DAMESHEK, 1962; GOOD and GABRIELSEN, 1964;
DEFENDI and METCALF, 1964; MILLER and DUKOR, 1964; METCALF, 1966;
WOLSTENHOLME and PORTER, 1966).

It appears worthwhile to again critically review present information on
thymic function(s) with emphasis on the development and maintenance of
immunologic competence. Results obtained in a systematic study in one
strain of specific pathogen-free mice will be reported. Critical comparison
of these findings with those of other workers clearly points out the following: 1) it may be hazardous to study the effects of neonatal thymectomy on
immune mechanisms in animals which were not raised in a specific patho-

gen-free or germfree environment; 2) as a prerequisite for interpretation of thymectomy results more information is needed on the kinetics and growth characteristics of the thymus involved; and 3) interpretative comparisons of findings in different species and extrapolations to clinical situations in man may lead to fallacious conclusions when established facts are not clearly distinguished from hypothetical propositions.

2. Phylogenetic and Ontogenetic Considerations

All expressions of acquired immunity, such as humoral antibody formation, immediate and delayed hypersensitivity, and transplantation immunity, are based on the organism's ability to a) specifically recognize antigenic determinants, b) actively produce specific protein molecules, and c) develop mechanisms by which the antigen may be recognized in anamnestic situations. These specialized reactions appear to depend on the normal development and function of a lymphoreticular system.

2.1. Phylogeny of Acquired Immunity

The phylogenetic development of the lymphoreticular system and of acquired immunity has been studied since the turn of the century (METCHNIKOFF, 1902); extensive reviews have appeared recently (see GOOD and PAPERMASTER, 1964).

In invertebrates, no evidence of acquired immunity, in the sense outlined above, has been observed. It should be noted, however, that some degree of recognition of foreignness could be demonstrated in the earthworm *(Lumbricus terrestris)* by CAMERON (1932) who found that homologous spermatozoa remained within the coelomic cavity considerably longer than heterologous (rabbit) spermatozoa or human erythrocytes; METALNIKOV and GASCHEN (1920) observed in caterpillars increased phagocytosis of, and development of resistance to, bacteria against which they had been "immunized"; we ignore, however, if these phenomena are based on a truly acquired capacity of the individual and if they represent specific processes in the sense of immunologic specificity. PHILLIPS (1960) reported on the formation of reactive, "antibody-like" substances in invertebrates following contact with antigens such as bovine serum albumine or coliphage. These findings are remarkable since lymphoreticular structures or organs have not been observed in invertebrates, although CAMERON (1934) had labeled some of the cells of the hemolymph "lymphocytes". It appears that invertebrates have to rely exclusively on enzymatic and phagocytotic mechanisms in their defense against pathogens (CANTACUZÈNE, 1923; BAER, 1944; BISSET, 1947; GOOD and PAPERMASTER, 1964; ROOS, 1967).

Early studies on manifestations of immunity in vertebrates were mostly concerned with the reaction to pathogens and the development of resistance upon reinfection (METCHNIKOFF, 1902). Humoral antibody formation was demonstrated in teleost fishes, and the finding of GEE and SMITH (1941) that trout could be actively immunized with killed organisms of *Bacteria salmonicida* may have been of economic interest. Anaphylaxis in teleost fish could be elicited by two spaced intraperitoneal injections of horse serum (DREYER and KING, 1948). HILDEMANN (1957, 1961) reviewed most of the earlier reports on transplantation experiments in lower vertebrates, and he was able to show that goldfish *(Carassius auratus)* rejected a second set of scale homografts with typical signs of a second-set reaction. The phylogenetic development of lymphoreticular tissue in lower vertebrates was widely unknown until GOOD and his associates reviewed and extended research on the phylogeny of immune reactions in vertebrates (GOOD and PAPERMASTER, 1964; GOOD et al., 1966; FINSTAD and GOOD, 1966).

The most primitive representative of vertebrates studied were the cyclostomes, the California hagfish *(Eptatretus stoutii)* and the sea lamprey *(Petromyzon marinus)*. In two hagfish species, hemopoietic foci were found in the lamina propria of the gut and in an organ derived from the anterior kidney; in these animals neither a thymus, nor lymphoid foci, nor plasma cells could be found. A circulating mononuclear cell, morphologically similar to a small lymphocyte, may be instrumental in inflammatory responses following injection of Freund's adjuvant (FINSTAD and GOOD, 1966). No signs of acquired immunity were demonstrable, and hagfish were found to be lacking in gammaglobulins (PAPERMASTER et al., 1962 a). The lamprey has a more organized hemopoietic systems, localized in the gill region, in a primitive marrow, and in the spleen. A rudimentary thymus, composed of foci of lymphoid cells, may be found in the region of the pharyngeal pouches (SALKIND, 1915). The circulating blood, the spleen and the marrow contain lymphocytes, but plasma cells are not present. Lampreys are able to reject homografts and to exhibit delayed hypersensitivity reactions to tuberculin. Among a variety of antigens tested, only *Brucella* antigens were able to elicit agglutinin formation in most animals; responses to hemocyanin and T2 coliphage were feeble or absent, and no antibody formation was observed following stimulation with bovine albumin, bovine gamma globulin, diphtheria toxoid, sheep red cells, rabbit red cells, or *Salmonella typhi* H- and O-antigens (FINSTAD and GOOD, 1966).

A well-developed thymus, with clear separation into cortex and medulla, was found in lower elasmobranchs (guitarfish, *Rhinobatos productus,* and horned shark, *Heterodontus francisci*). Authentic lymphoid tissue was present in the spleen, the lamina propria of the gut, and in the parenchyma of the kidneys; plasma cells were absent. These lower elasmobranchs, although unable to produce antibody against bovine serum albumin, responded to such antigens as hemocyanin, T2 coliphage and *Brucella*, and rejected skin homografts (FINSTAD and GOOD, 1966); vigorous antibody formation following stimulation with PR-8 influenza virus could be elicited in the lemonshark *(Negaprion brevirostris)* (SIGEL and CLEM, 1963). In higher sharks and rays the lymphoid tissue is developed to a similar degree; whereas in rays no definite plasma cells were found in the spleen, mature plasma cells were observed in sharks (GOOD et al., 1966).

The paddlefish *(Polyodon spathula)*, as a representative chondrostean, the bowfin *(Amia calva)*, as a representative holostean, and several teleosts all possess thymic tissue, a well-developed spleen with plasma cells, and gut-associated lymphoid foci.

Table 1. *Phylogenetic development of the lymphoid system and of acquired immunity in fishes* (GOOD et al., *1966*)

	Lymphoid system	Immunologic Competence
Hagfish	Primitive lymphoid hemoblasts	
Lamprey	Lymphoid cells in pharyngeal epithelium, Primitive spleen, Circulating lymphocytes	Delayed hypersensitivity, Homograft immunity (Antibody responses, immunologic memory, immunoglobulins?)
Hornshark Guitarfish	Definite thymus and spleen	Humoral antibody responses, Complex immunoglobulins
Elasmobranchs Chondrosteans Holosteans Teleosts	Plasma cells	Definite primary and secondary immune responses

In amphibians primitive nodules, composed of lymphoid cells, may be found in the sublingual region, but only in reptiles and higher vertebrates are the tonsils lymphoepithelial structures with a clear separation into different zones, and for the first time in the evolutionary scale, plasma cells are found in the lamina propria of the gut.

The development of the bursa of Fabricius as a gut-associated lymphoepithelial organ in birds appears to be a unique step in evolution. The bursa, together with the thymus, plays an important role in the establishment of immunologic competence in the developing bird (GLICK et al., 1956; WARNER et al., 1962; COOPER et al., 1965).

Studies on the lymphoid tissues of the Australian echidna *(Tachyglossus aculeatus)* revealed that this very primitive representative of the mammals possesses a bilobed thymus, spleen, appendix, tonsillar tissue and numerous lymph nodules, each consisting of a single follicle; no Peyer's patches could be found. This animal appears to be unable to produce antibodies following stimulation with sheep red cells or bovine serum albumin; antibody formation after immunization with *Salmonella adelaide* flagellar antigen was measurable, but the titers obtained were considerably lower than those elicited in mice or rats (DIENER and EALEY, 1965). In mammals no bursa can be found, and attempts to clearly define a bursa-equivalent tissue have failed so far. GOOD and his collaborators (see COOPER et al., 1967) propose that some of the gut-associated lymphoid tissue in mammals, including Peyer's patches, appendix and sacculus rotundus in rabbits, and the tonsils, may have a function similar to the one ascribed to the bursa in birds. It will become apparent that many inconsistencies have to be resolved before this hypothesis can be accepted.

These phylogenetic studies suggest, as summarized in Table 1, a dependence of the development of immunologic capacity on the evolution of the thymus and other lymphoreticular structures.

2.2. Ontogenetic Development of the Lymphoreticular Tissue and of Acquired Immunity

The sequence of the phylogenetic development of the lymphoreticular system is, in part, reflected in the ontogenesis of mammals. During embryogenesis of all mammalian species studied so far, the thymus is the first lymphoid organ to be recognized as such (BEARD, 1900; HAMMAR, 1905; DE WINIWATER, 1933; KAY et al., 1962; LA VIA et al., 1963; KELLY, 1963; BLOCK, 1964; ARCHER et al., 1964 a; ADNER et al., 1965). The mammalian thymus appears to grow out ventrally from the third and fourth branchial pouches as paired epithelial evaginations.

The following details about further development of the thymus pertain to the sequence of events described in mice but may apply also to other species. The primitive thymus migrates caudally to reach the pericardium and remains purely epithelial until the 12th day of intrauterine life. It has been established that the first lymphopoietic activity can be detected in mouse embryonic thymus by the 14th day of gestation, and that at 16 days the organ has become primarily lymphoid (BALL and AUERBACH, 1960; GOOD and PAPERMASTER, 1964; KÖBBERLING, 1965); the newborn mouse has circulating lymphocytes and diffuse accumulations of lymphoid cells in the spleen (MILLER, 1964 a). Of great importance is the fact that in germfree animals the thymus, even after birth, remains the only major lymphoid organ, the lymphoid tissue of other sites remaining poorly developed (GORDON, 1959).

Whereas these findings of descriptive embryology have never been disputed, controversy arose early concerning the mechanisms by which the primarily epithelial structure of the thymus changes to assume its lymphoid appearance. On the one hand, it has been postulated that thymic lymphocytes are of mesodermal origin, the progeny of mesenchymal cells which had migrated into the epithelial thymus anlage ("immigration theory") (HAMMAR, 1905; MAXIMOW, 1909; BADERTSCHER, 1915; KINGSBURY, 1915). On the other hand, MAURER (1886) and STÖHR (1906, 1910) claimed that thymocytes arose by transformation directly from the epithelial cells. Other followers of this "transformation theory" included DUSTIN (1913) and GRÉGOIRE (1932). DE WINIWATER (1933) chose an intermediate stand between the two opposing viewpoints and proposed that thymic lymphocytes arose from the epithelial anlage in early embryogenesis of the guinea pig but that in later stages of development immigrating cells could also serve as progenitor cells of thymocytes. More recently, AUERBACH and his associates attempted an experimental approach to this problem which could not be resolved on purely morphological grounds.

AUERBACH's findings, recently reviewed (AUERBACH, 1964 a, b; 1966), were obtained in intricate *in vitro* experiments performed on embryonic mouse tissue fragments (AUERBACH, 1960, 1961 a, b). The trypsin-treated thymus of a 12-day old mouse embryo remained epithelial when grown in tissue culture (BALL and AUERBACH, 1960). However, lymphoid cells appeared in the epithelial thymus when it was transplanted into the anterior chamber of the eye of an adult mouse. Epithelial thymic fragments, obtained after tryptic treatment of 12-day old embryonic organs, also were observed to become lymphoid in tissue culture when grown in close contact with mesenchyme of different sources (salivary gland, lung, kidney, etc.) (AUERBACH, 1960, 1964 a, b). These findings were interpreted by Auerbach as strong evidence for the direct transformation of epithelial thymus cells into lymphoid cells in the mouse; the transformation is thought to be induced by a mesenchymal stimulus on the epithelial thymus anlage. The epithelium, according to AUERBACH (1966), would be the main, if not the only, source of lymphoid cells during embryogenesis of the thymus. AUERBACH's hypotheses have so far not been confirmed by kinetic studies using stable cell markers.

In a series of electron-microscopic studies, ACKERMAN and KNOUFF (1959, 1964) and ACKERMANN (1962) came to the conclusion that in birds a similar transformation of the epithelial bursa anlage into a lymphoid organ occurred under the influence of mesenchymal contact. It would be desirable to have these morphological findings also corroborated by kinetic studies.

The appearance of lymphoid elements in lymph nodes, in the spleen, and in the peripheral blood was shown to be secondary in time to the lymphoid development of the thymus (BEARD, 1900; HAMMAR, 1905, 1921; RUTH,

1960; KAY et al., 1962; LA VIA et al., 1963). The origin of these extrathymic lymphocytes, and the possible role played in their appearance by the thymus, are largely unknown. Because pertinent evidence based on kinetic experiments is lacking, discussion on this question remains highly speculative. AUERBACH (1963, 1966) did not observe lymphoid transformation in cultures of spleen rudiments from 13- to 14-day old mouse embryos or in bone marrow from femur fragments of 15- to 17-day old mouse embryos. When spleen or bone marrow rudiments were grown in contact with embryonic thymus, lymphoid cells were seen in both spleen and bone marrow; this effect was also observed when the two tissues were separated by a Millipore membrane. Evidence for the thymic origin of lymphoid cells proliferating in the spleen was obtained in a complex *in vitro* experiment. When 9-day old embryonic chick spleen was cultured together with embryonic mouse thymus, the lymphoid elements in the spleen could bei identified as mouse cells; when in a combined culture of embryonic mouse spleen and thymus rudiments the tissues were separated by a Millipore membrane, lymphoid cells appeared in the thymus but not in the spleen (AUERBACH, 1964 a).

The present views as expressed by AUERBACH (1964 a), MILLER and DAVIES (1964) and others, on the ontogeny of the lymphoid system may be summarized as follows: 1) primary lymphoid anlagen develop in the thymus by transformation of epithelial elements under the influence of a mesenchymal induction mechanism; 2) most or all lymphoid cells in early embryogenesis may be formed within the primitive thymus; and 3) these lymphoid cells may leave the embryonic thymus to populate the spleen and other lymphoid organs as precursors for lymphoid colonies.

One should not forget AUERBACH'S own statement (1964 a) that "there is no reason to assume, a priori, that a similar mechanism of cell origin applies to the functioning structure of the neonatal or adult animal". It may be pertinent to add an additional word of caution as to whether or not interpretations based on highly artificial *in vitro* experiments without the use of stable markers are 1) sufficient evidence for origin and transformation of cells, and 2) may be extrapolated to *in vivo* situations. For the understanding of a series of immunologic deficiency states in man it is of paramount importance to know if thymic epithelial cells do in fact give birth to lymphoid cells. This question has not been answered beyond doubt for *in vivo* conditions. The concept of an epithelial origin of all thymic lymphoid cells in early intrauterine life could not be reconciled with the assumption of a common precursor cell of extrathymic origin for both thymic and extrathymic, in particular gut-associated, lymphocytes (GOOD et al., 1967). There is a great need for kinetic studies performed on intact embryos and fetuses.

The time at which the developing organism achieves immunological competence has attracted much interest that goes back many years. In older observations (see GOOD and PAPERMASTER, 1964; SILVERSTEIN, 1964), most species were found to be nonresponsive to many antigens during prenatal development, and it was therefore believed that immunological responsiveness was acquired only at or after birth (OSBORN et al., 1952; SMITH and BRIDGES, 1958). Recent studies, however, presented evidence that some degree of immunologic capacity is present in some species already during embryonal or fetal life and in the neonatal period (SILVERSTEIN, 1964; STERZL and SILVERSTEIN, 1967).

Table 2. *Humoral antibody formation by fetal animals*

Species	Antigen	Age at which detectable antibody formed	Authors
Opossum (*Didelphys virginiana*)	Bacteriophage ΦX-174 *Salmonella typhi*	17-day-old pouch embryo [a] 8-day-old pouch embryo [a]	KALMUTZ, 1962 LA VIA et al., 1963
Quokka (*Setonix brachyurus*)	Sheep Red Cells	12- to 90-day-old pouch embryo [b]	STANLEY et al., 1966
Sheep	Bacteriophage ΦX-174 Ferritin Ovalbumin	35-day-old embryo 66-day-old embryo 125-day-old embryo	SILVERSTEIN, 1964
Pig	Actinophage MSP-9 *Escherichia coli* Hemocyanin	antibody formed against all 3 antigens when immunized at 3—5 days before birth	KIM et al., 1966 a, b
Calf	*Leptospira saxkoebing*	132- to 164-day-old embryo	FENNESTAD and BORG-PETERSON, 1962
Monkey	Ferritin Ovalbumin	120- to 180-day-old embryo	SILVERSTEIN and KRANER, 1965
Man	Maternal infection with *Toxoplasma* Rubella virus	non-maternal antibody in cordblood of infant	EICHENWALD and SHINEFELD, 1963 BAERLOCHER et al., 1967

[b] Leaves pouch at age 180 days   [a] Leaves pouch at age 60 days

Humoral antibody formation following stimulation with a variety of antigens could be elicited in many species before birth (Table 2). Fetal lambs were able to reject skin homografts at 85 days of gestation (SCHINCKEL and FERGUSON, 1953; SILVERSTEIN, 1964). Fetal rhesus monkeys could be effectively sensitized with homologous, adult bone marrow cells at the age of 9 weeks (BANGHAM et al., 1962). Evidence has been presented that the human fetus is capable of synthetizing IgG and IgM immunoglobulins as early as in the 20th week of gestation (VAN FURTH et al., 1965; KAY, 1967).

Studies on the development of humoral antibody formation in fetal lambs led SILVERSTEIN to propose that immunologic maturation may be a step-wise process during which the ability to respond to different antigens is acquired at different developmental stages (SILVERSTEIN, 1964; SILVERSTEIN et al., 1966): whereas the 35-day-old embryo readily produced antibody to bacteriophage ΦX-174 within a week after stimulation, the lamb was unable to form measurable amounts of antibody to *Salmonella typhi* or diphtheria toxoid up to the age of 6 weeks after birth.

While there is some evidence indicating that thymectomy in amphibian larvae interferes with skin graft rejection mechanisms (COOPER and HILDEMANN, 1965; DU PASQUIER, 1965), the linkage of the emergence of immune responsiveness to the development of the thymus and other lymphoid tissues could be most conveniently studied in marsupials. It has been shown in the opossum that antibody responses to bacteriophage ΦX-174 and *Salmonella typhi* could only be elicited at a time when thymus and lymph nodes contained lymphoid cells, but well before lymphoid cells had appeared in the spleen (KALMUTZ, 1962; LA VIA et al., 1963). In the Australian quokka, the development of an "external" and "internal" thymus has been noted (STANLEY et al., 1966). The mass of the external thymus, located bilaterally in the neck region, exceeds that of the internal thymus during most of the 180 days after birth the young spends in the pouch of the mother; at the time the young leaves the pouch, both external and internal thymus have approximately the same weight. Extirpation of the external thymus in the pouch embryo delayed the appearance of responsiveness to stimulation with sheep red cells, indicating that the external thymus may be necessary for the immunologic capacities of the quokka at that early age.

Research in the area of the ontogenetic development of immunity has only begun; more species should be studied and additional antigens should be used before the picture of the developmental biology of antibody production emerges more clearly.

3. Growth Characteristics and Cellular Kinetics of the Thymus

The thymus has been found to be the site of most intensive lymphopoiesis in young animals of many mammalian species examined (BEARD, 1900; KINDRED, 1940, 1942; ANDREASEN and OTTESEN, 1944; ANDREASEN and CHRISTENSEN, 1949; FICHTELIUS, 1960; BIERRING, 1960; METCALF, 1964). On the basis of the number of mitotic figures in the thymus of young and adult rats, KINDRED (1940, 1942) and ANDREASEN and CHRISTENSEN (1949) estimated that more lymphoid cells were produced than would be necessary to sustain the rate of thymic growth. Only recently these estimates have been substantiated by kinetic studies in which the incorporation of tritiated thymidine into newly synthetized DNA was followed autoradiographically (COTTIER, 1964, 1966; METCALF and WIADROWSKI, 1966; MICHALKE et al., 1967). Although it has never been questioned that lymphoid cells leave the thymus, the magnitude of this emigration is subject to controversy. The following two possibilities are under discussion:

1. a substantial number of lymphoid cells constantly leaves the thymus, this emigration being higher in the young as opposed to the adult organism (COTTIER, 1965; ERNSTRÖM et al., 1965; ERNSTRÖM and LARSSON, 1966; KOTANI et al., 1966; LINNA, 1967 a, b; MICHALKE et al., 1967; WEISSMAN, 1967), or

2. a vast majority of the newly produced lymphoid cells die in the thymus while only few cells ever leave the organ (see METCALF, 1966 a, b).

For our understanding of the effects of thymectomy performed during the perinatal period of life, further studies are needed on the fate of thymic lymphoid cells at that particular time; it would be of interest to know what number of thymic lymphoid cells does actually leave the thymus per unit time. A meaningful assessment of these processes requires more information on at least the following parameters as a function of age before and after birth: 1) rate of thymic growth; 2) proliferative activity of thymic lymphoid cells with a meaningful estimate of the generation or cell cycle time of the majority of these cells; and 3) a quantitative estimate of intrathymic cell loss.

3.1. Growth Characteristics of the Thymus

While the postnatal growth of the thymus has been studied in several species, information on thymic growth rates in the prenatal period is scarce. In a detailed study, KAY et al. (1962) recorded the thymic weights of 289 human fetuses of different ages. While the thymic growth curve obtained reflected an almost linear weight increase throughout most of intrauterine life, the rate of growth diminished at the beginning of the third trimester (25 to 28 weeks). This change in growth rate was not emphasized since the authors felt it might have been caused by a series of accidental factors (premature births, infection, etc.). A similar biphasic curve with the indication of a change in the thymic growth rate around birth was obtained in mice by BALL (1963) who registered the total number of thymic lymphoid cells in animals of different age groups with the aid of a Coulter counter. BALL found an approximately ten-fold increase in the total lymphoid cell mass between 4 and 2 days before birth; after a short stationary period around the time of birth, the total number of thymic cells increased about five-fold between 2 and 14 days after birth.

In order to obtain more detailed information on the growth of mouse thymus during the perinatal period of life, wet thymic weights were recorded of a total of 260 BNL-Swiss mice (Hale-Stoner strain); the age of the mice ranged from 4 days before to 6 days after birth (COTTIER, 1966; HESS et al., 1967).

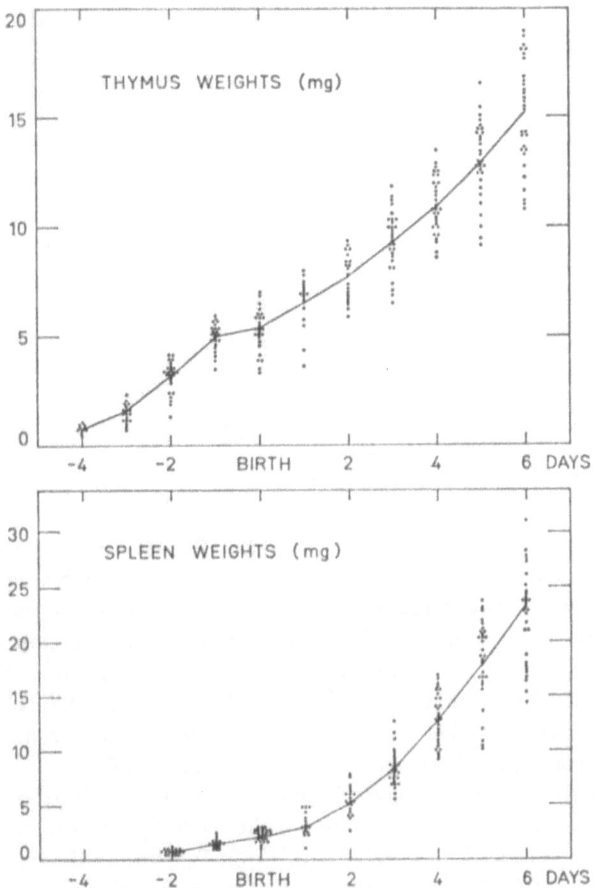

Fig. 1. Wet thymus and spleen weights of BNL-Swiss mice in relation to age

As evident from Fig. 1 thymic weights increased at a steady rate up to the age of 1½ to 1 day before birth. From then on, a diminished rate of thymic weight increase was noted. Statistical analysis by calculation of linear regressions revealed that before birth thymic weight increased daily by a factor of 1.9 while the daily relative weight gain after birth was only 1.2. The difference between the two slopes was shown to be highly significant ($P < 0.001$). A growth curve of body weights recorded in mice of similar age groups is presented in Fig. 2; linear regressions could not be calculated from this curve so that the increases in body and thymic weight could not be directly compared.

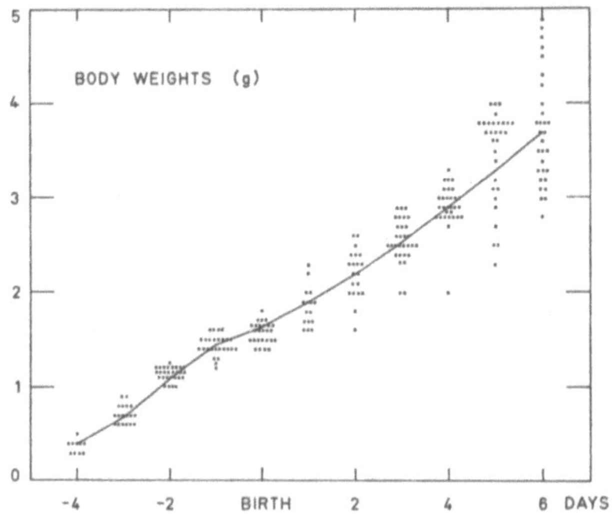

Fig. 2. Body weights of BNL-Swiss mice in relation to age

This observation of a prenatal change in the rate of thymic growth in mice is consistent with and extends the earlier findings of KAY et al. (1962) and BALL (1963). The break in the weight curve of the thymus could be explained by 1) a change in the degree of migration of cells out of the thymus, 2) a change in the mean generation time of proliferating thymic lymphoid cells, 3) a diminished influx of cells, 4) a rate of intrathymic cell death after birth greather than before birth, or 5) two or more of these possibilities combined (COTTIER, 1966; HESS et al., 1967).

After birth the thymic weight in mice increases steadily to reach a maximum in terms of ratio of thymus weight to body weight at the age of 2 weeks (AXELRAD and VAN DER GAAG, 1962; WILSON et al., 1964 a; MILLER and DUKOR, 1964). In sheep, the relative thymic weight is highest at the time of birth, while in man this maximum is reached already during the 25th to 28th week of gestation (KAY et al., 1962). After that peak a relative regression of the weight of the thymus was noted in all mammalian species.

It should be noted that in a direct comparison of thymic growth and regression rates of germfree and conventional CFW mice, WILSON et al. (1964 a) noted a significant difference: the thymus of conventional mice grew at a much faster rate than the thymus of germfree animals during the first two weeks of postnatal life; no significant difference in thymic weights was observed after the age of one month. This finding is not easily reconciled with the notion that thymic growth occurs independent of antigenic stimulation (METCALF, 1964).

3.2. Proliferation of Thymic Lymphoid Cells

The relative proliferative activity of thymic lymphoid cells in terms of overall mitotic indices is from 5 to 10 times higher than that observed in all lymphoid cells of spleen, Peyer's patches or lymph nodes (ANDREASEN and CHRISTENSEN, 1949; METCALF, 1964).

Since most of the studies on the proliferative activity of thymic lymphoid cells were carried out either in intact young adult animals (CRADDOCK et al., 1964; EVERETT et al., 1964; METCALF, 1964; METCALF and WIADROWSKI, 1966) or in thymus grafts from donors of various age groups (METCALF, 1964; MATSUYAMA et al., 1966), it appeared of interest to examine proliferating thymic lymphoid cells in intact mice during the immediate pre- and postnatal period of life (HESS et al., 1967; MICHALKE et al., 1967).

The overall proliferative activity was estimated autoradiographically by the initial incorporation of tritiated thymidine in thymic lymphoid cells. BNL-Swiss mice were given single injections of tritiated thymidine at from 3 days before birth to 6 days after birth. Smears of thymic tissue were made 30 minutes after administration of the tritiated DNA precursor; an average of 4,000 lymphoid cells was evaluated for each age group, and mitotic figures were recorded separately.

Results are presented in Fig. 3. It may be seen that the relative number of proliferating cells reached a peak at between 3 and 4 days after birth, as evident from coinciding significant increases in 1) the number of mitotic figures per thousand cells, and 2) the overall initial labeling index after injection of tritiated thymidine. At the time of this proliferative peak an increase in the relative number of medium and large lymphoid cells with a corresponding drop in the relative number of small lymphocytes was observed. Even when taking into account several sources of autoradiographic error (COTTIER et al., 1964 b), it appeared justified to state that a greater number of thymic lymphoid cells was actively proliferating at 3 and 4 days after birth than at any time during the observation period. The fact that thymic weight increased at a steady rate during the entire postnatal period indicates either massive migration of cells out of the thymus or equally massive cell death within the thymus at around day 3 to 4 after birth.

For an estimate of the cell cycle time of thymic lymphoid cells, MICHALKE et al. (1967) examined labeling index and labeling intensity of mitotic figures in the thymus of 2-day-old BNL-Swiss mice. The animals were sacrificed at from 10 minutes to 24 hours after a single intraperitoneal injection of tritiated thymidine.

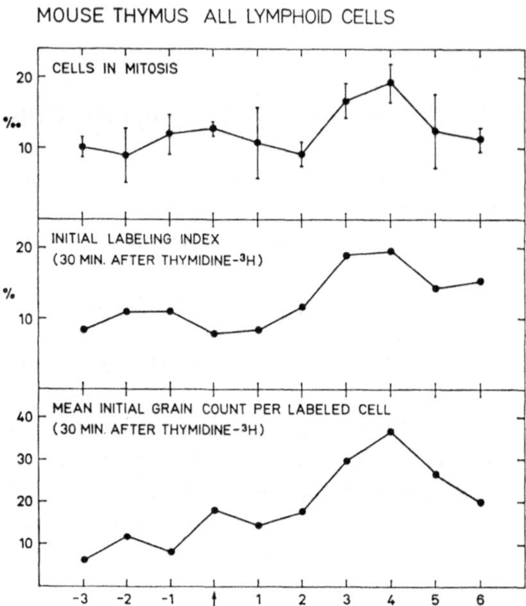

Fig. 3. Proliferative pattern of BNL-Swiss thymic lymphoid cells in relation to age. Top: Number of mitotic figures per 1,000 lymphoid cells. Middle: Initial labeling indices of thymic lymphoid cells. Progressive background correction: > 1 = two and more grains; > 2 = three and more grains; > 3 = four and more grains; > 4 = five and more grains. Bottom: Mean grain counts of initially labeled thymic lymphoid cells (four and more grains). (By permission of *Nature*)

The percentage of labeled mitotic figures (MLI = mitotic labeling index) of thymic lymphoid cells is plotted in Fig. 4 as a function of the time interval between thymidine injection and sacrifice. A steep rise in the MLI is observed in mice sacrificed between 80 and 110 minutes after administration of tritiated thymidine, and the MLI remains between 90 and 100% in preparations obtained in the 2- to 8-hour intervals. At between 8 to 9 hours after thymidine injection a sharp drop in the MLI curve may be noted. An abortive second peak is reached at the 17-hour interval.

From their data MICHALKE et al. (1967) were able to estimate the following approximative durations of cell cycle phases of dividing lymphoid cells in the thymus of 2-day-old mice:

1. Duration of G_2 (= time interval between the end of DNA synthesis and onset of prophase) was calculated at from 35 to 48 minutes for a small group of cells; the duration of G_2 for the majority of thymic lymphoid cells, however, was found to be in the order of from 86 to 94 minutes.

2. *Duration of M* (= mitosis) may range from 27 to 44 minutes or less for the majority of cells. While, therefore, the total duration of $G_2 + M$ may be as short as 62 minutes for a small group of cells, for the majority of cells a time of from 113 to 138 minutes appeared to be a reasonable estimate.

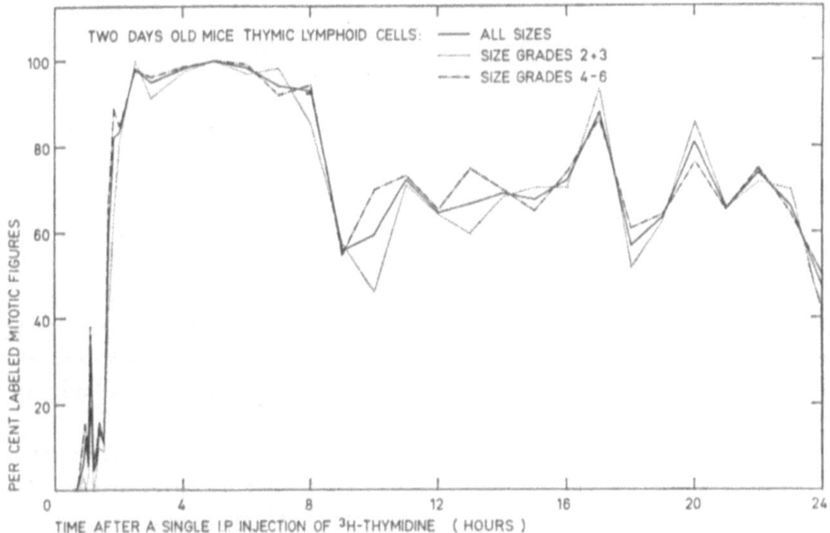

Fig. 4. Number of labeled thymic lymphoid cells in mitosis as a function of time after a single injection of ³H-thymidine

3. *Duration of S* (= DNA synthesis phase) was found to be 6¹/₂ to 7¹/₂ hours for the majority of cells.

4. The best estimate for the *total generation time* of most lymphoid cells in the thymus was 9 to 9¹/₂ hours.

5. *Duration of G_1* (= time interval between the end of mitosis and onset of DNA synthesis) could not be calculated directly on the basis of these data. Subtraction of the proposed estimates for the duration of $S + G_2 + M$ from the generation time of 9 to 9¹/₂ hours leaves only a short time for the duration of G_1 .

Generation times of medium and large thymic lymphoid cells were not markedly different.

These findings in newborn mice differ from results reported by METCALF and WIADROWSKI (1966) who studied the proliferative activity of thymic lymphoid cells in 2-month-old AKR mice. On the basis of mean grain count halfing times following a single injection of tritiated thymidine, these authors calculated a total duration of G_2+M of 78 minutes, a duration of S of 5½ hours, and a mean cell cycle time of 6.8 hours for large and of 8.2 hours for medium-sized lymphoid cells. It should be emphasized, however, as previously discussed by JANETT et al. (1966), that it is hazardous to base the determination of the generation time of lymphoid cells on mean grain count halfing times since mean grain counts of interphase cells do not follow a simple exponential function after the injection of tritiated thymidine.

Under the assumption that the difference between generation times of thymic lymphoid cells of newborn and adult mice is real, this observation may indicate a change in the proliferation pattern of lymphoid cells of the thymus with advancing age. Immigration of cells into the newborn thymus was found to be absent or very low (GOWANS, 1964), while a greater percentage of cells, maybe with shorter generation times, appear to immigrate into the thymus of adult animals (HARRIS and FORD, 1964; FORD, 1966). In none of these experiments demonstrating immigration of lymphoid cells into the thymus has it been indicated in which thymic zone these migrant cells lodge. The exact route of entry and the subsequent fate of immigrating cells have to be established in an anatomically intact thymus before the significance of this immigration and the particular role of these migrant cells may be evaluated.

In a recent study BRUMBY and METCALF (1967) joined C57BL or AKR mice in parabiosis. While the blood flow between partners was arrested for one hour by clamping, one of the parabionts was given a single injection of tritiated thymidine. Three days after release of the clamp, labeled migrant cells were found in the thymus of the noninjected mouse to be localized mainly in the medulla or at the cortico-medullary junction. This finding indicates that immigrating cells, under these conditions, may follow intrathymic routes different from those of cells produced in the thymic cortex. In view of the fact that lymphoid cells of the thymic cortex represent both a more homogenous and more primitive population of cells than lymph node lymphocytes, as judged by nucleolar size and cytoplasmic volume and differentiation (HEINIGER et al., 1967), it should be particularly rewarding to separately study both fate and immunologic potential of thymic cortical and medullary lymphoid cells.

3.3. Intrathymic Fate of Newly Produced Lymphoid Cells

In relating the number of mitotic cells to various thymic zones, it became evident that most dividing cells were located in the outer half of the thymic cortex while the number of mitotic cells in the medulla was relatively small (METCALF, 1964; HINRICHSEN, 1964; KÖBBERLING, 1965; LINNA and STILLSTRÖM, 1966; MICHALKE et al., 1967).

The percentage of initially labeling lymphoid cells in the thymus of fetal and newborn mice (KÖBBERLING, 1965) and of adult mice (HINRICHSEN, 1965) was followed autoradiographically after a single injection of tritiated thymidine. Heavily labeled cells were detected in the outer zone of the thymic cortex as early as from 15 to 30 minutes after thymidine injection; labeling of cells located in the inner zone of the cortex and in the medulla was negligible at that period of time. A gradual shift in labeling intensity was observed: the number of labeled cells of the inner cortical zone and of the medulla started to increase at from one to two hours after the injection of tritiated thymidine to reach a maximum at 12 to 24 hours. At the time of maximum labeling of the medullary lymphoid cells the number of labeled cells in the outer cortex started to decrease. These findings indicate a migration of cells from the outer cortical zones of the thymus to the medulla, in confirmation of earlier reports by METCALF (1964).

Radiochemical and autoradiographic studies following systemic or local labeling of thymic lymphoid cells with tritiated thymidine appear to show that newly formed cells spend from 2 to 4 days within the thymus of rats (CRADDOCK et al., 1964; EVERETT et al., 1964), mice (METCALF, 1966 b), and guinea pigs (LINNA and STILLSTRÖM, 1966). According to hypothetical models proposed by SAINTE-MARIE and LEBLOND (1965) and METCALF (1966 b) small medullary lymphoid cells are the progeny of large "stem" cells located in the thymic cortex. These models should be regarded with extreme caution since exceptions to the concept that small lymphoid cells are derived from medium-sized lymphocytes which in turn are the progeny of large cells have been reported (CRONKITE, 1967).

3.3.1. Intrathymic Cell Death

METCALF (1966 a, b) believes that at the end of their intrathymic lifespan most of the newly produced small lymphocytes disintegrate within the thymus. Supposedly this breakdown of thymic lymphocytes is an explosive process which, according to METCALF and BRUMBY (1966) might be linked to and mediated by the action of cortisone; this assumption was necessitated by the fact that the number of pyknotic cells (NAKAMURA and METCALF, 1961) is too small to account for massive cell death (COTTIER, 1966; MICHALKE et al., 1967; SCHAEDELI et al., 1967).

3.3.2. Migration of Lymphoid Cells from the Thymus

KINDRED (1942) postulated that from 80 to 90% of thymic lymphoid cells leave the organ. Direct evidence for massive thymic cell migration to peripheral lymphoid organs, however, was lacking because methods for its detection were not available.

2*

FICHTELIUS (1958) who labeled rat thymic lymphoid cells *in vitro* with ^{32}P and infused them intravenously into other rats, found ^{32}P-labeled DNA localized mainly in the spleen. Autoradiography of lymphoid organs from guinea pigs following transfusion of thymic cells which were labeled with ^{32}P or tritiated thymidine revealed that these transfused cells were located in the perifollicular regions of the spleen and of lymph nodes (DIDERHOLM and FICHTELIUS, 1959; DIDERHOLM, 1961). Since this distribution of label was not observed after the transfusion of dead cells, it was assumed that the observed radioactivity was associated with living cells.

In a different approach, HARRIS and FORD (1963) thymectomized either CBA/H or CBA/H-T6T6 mice after birth and grafted the thymectomized animals at the age of 7 to 8 days with newborn thymic tissue from the other strain. The animals were sacrificed at from 4 to 12 weeks after grafting. In 27-day-old recipients a maximum of 65% of donor-type mitoses was identified in lymph nodes. The number of migrant lymphoid cells in lymph nodes started to decrease substantially at 6 weeks after thymus implantation, and no dividing donor cells were detected beyond the 80-day interval. It was concluded that under these conditions thymus lymphoid cells may selectively migrate to and proliferate in lymph nodes; the possibility was also considered that after a certain time thymic grafts might release immigrated host cells. This latter possibility was tested in an experiment in which neonatally thymectomized mice were used as primary and secondary hosts for newborn thymus grafts from donors with two, one or no chromosome marker. A measurable number of cells, derived from the primary host, was observed to be released from the thymus graft and to migrate to lymph nodes when the graft was placed in a secondary host (HARRIS and FORD, 1964). Only few lymphoid cells from the thymus could be traced to the spleen or bone marrow of either primary or secondary host. This latter finding is in contrast to the observation of MILLER (1962 b) who, in neonatally thymectomized 10- to 18-week-old (Ak×T6)F$_1$ mice, grafted at one week of age with either a newborn Ak or C3H thymus, regularly found about 20% of the dividing spleen cells to be of donor origin. Similar results were also reported by LEUCHARS et al. (1965).

In contrast, MATSUYAMA et al. (1966) who studied the proliferation of multiple neonatal thymic grafts in adult C57BL mice came to the conclusion that only few, if any, lymphoid cells ever leave the thymus. Within two weeks after a single intravenous injection of tritiated thymidine, the percentage of labeled blood lymphocytes or lymphoid cells of subcutaneous or mesenteric lymph nodes did not increase above the initially observed level of 10%; labeling indices of both the animal's own thymus and thymus grafts had risen to 90% already at 3 days after thymidine injection. Based on the assumption that thymic lymphocytes were regenerated every 3 to 4 days, it was estimated that fewer than 0.5% of the newly formed lymphocytes could have seeded to the host lymphoid tissues within 3 and 6 days after labeling.

Neither cell transfer studies nor experiments with transplanted thymic tissue truly reflect the situation in the intact animal. The integrity of lymph vessels appears to be of particular importance for free passage of cells out of the thymus; this prerequisite almost certainly is not met even in a fully vascularized graft.

KOTANI et al. (1966) canulated the efferent duct of the right cervical lymph node in adult guinea pigs and measured the difference in the lymphocyte output before and after ablation of the right thymic lobe. A daily output of 12×10^6 lymphoid cells from both thymic lobes was calculated which would represent 12% of the total number of circulating lymphocytes. In young adult guinea pigs, ERNSTRÖM et al. (1965) and ERNSTRÖM and LARSSON (1966) compared the relative content of lymphocytes in blood from the right carotid artery, close to the origin of the right thymic artery, with that of blood obtained from either the right thymic vein or a femoral vein. The percentage of lymphocytes in the thymic vein was higher than in either carotid artery or femoral vein, thus indicating a contribution of lymphocytes by the thymus.

The possibility of lymphocyte migration from the thymus has also been studied autoradiographically following direct local labeling of the thymus. NOSSAL (1964) and NOSSAL and GORRIE (1964) instilled a total of 20 μc of tritiated thymidine with a "high specific activity" either by punction of the thymic artery or by diffuse microinfiltration under the thymic capsule into newborn or adult guinea pigs. Animals were sacrificed at one hour and then every day up to 7 days after the administration of tritiated thymidine. A initial labeling index of 10% was observed at the one-hour interval; the labeled cells were mostly medium-sized lymphocytes located in the outer thymic cortex. At 4 days after the injection of the tritiated thymidine, about 50% of all thymic lymphocytes were labeled, but mean grain counts were "very low" at that time. The relative number of cells, presumably coming from the thymus, could be identified in lymph nodes by mean grain counts many times higher than mean grain counts attributable to reutilization of tritiated DNA or nucleotides. The percentage of the lymphoid cells thus identified as migrant cells in mesenteric lymph nodes of adult guinea pigs rose from 0.4% at day 1 to 11% at day 4 after the administration of tritiated thymidine. In contrast, about 8 to 10 times as many migrant cells were found in mesenteric lymph nodes of newborn animals. NOSSAL calculated that a maximum of one in every 50 "new" cell in the mesenteric lymph node may be thymus-derived; the discrepancy between this estimate and the high mitotic activity of the thymus was interpreted as suggestive of intrathymic death of a large proportion of newly formed thymic lymphocytes. Essentially similar results were obtained by MURRAY and WOODS (1964).

These estimates are probably too low due to limitations inherent in the autoradiographic technique. Evidence for massive migration of lymphoid cells from the thymus in 2-day-old mice has been obtained by the following approach. Thymic weights of BNL-Swiss mice were observed to increase by 14.3% from day 2 to day 3 after birth while during the same period of time the percentage of initially labeling lymphoid cells increased from 12 to 19% (HESS et al., 1967). It was estimated that the duration of DNA synthesis was covering from 72 to 78% of the total duration of the cell cycle of most thymic lymphoid cells (MICHALKE et al., 1967). Based on a comparison of this estimate with initial labeling indices it may be calculated that almost one-third of the total number of lymphoid cells in the thymus may be newly produced during this particular 24-hour-interval. Since the mean increment of thymic weight during the same interval is only 14.3%, migration of cells out of the thymus and/or intrathymic cell death would have to account for the difference. Pyknotic cells as evidence for intrathymic cell death are very rare at 2 days after birth (SCHAEDELI et al., 1967), so that a large percentage of thymic lymphoid cells presumably leaves the organ.

These conclusions are strongly supported by recent experiments in which the distribution of tritiated DNA in different lymphoid organs was measured radiochemically following local labeling of thymic cells with tritiated thymidine (LINNA and STILLSTRÖM, 1966; LINNA, 1967 a, b; WEISSMAN, 1967). Taking into consideration most of the known sources of error due to a direct labeling procedure, a significant transport of thymus cell DNA to the spleen of young adult guinea pigs was evident at 48 hours after the administration of tritiated thymidine (LINNA and STILLSTRÖM, 1966). Since no definite localization of label was observed after transfusion of labeled dead lymphoid cells (DIDERHOLM, 1961), and since the labeling pattern of lymphoid organs following intrathymic labeling was significantly different from that obtained after systemic labeling, LINNA postulated that the measured radioactivity was associated with DNA of living cells. In young rabbits, highest levels of ^{3}H-DNA derived from thymic cells could also be demonstrated in the spleen, whereas lower but still significant amounts were present in mesenteric lymph nodes, bone marrow and tonsils (LINNA, 1967 a). Autoradiography and radiochemical determination of ^{3}H-DNA following intrathymic labeling with tritiated thymidine were combined for the evaluation of thymic cell migration in 5-day-old, 21-day-old and several months old hamsters (LINNA, 1967 b). Heavily labeled lymphoid cells were found at 2 days after thymidine injection in mesenteric lymph nodes of one-week-old animals while none could be detected in the spleen which at this stage of development still contains only very few lymphocytes. In 3-week-old hamsters, thymic migrant cells were present in mesenteric lymph nodes, spleen and Peyer's patches; only few migrant lymphoid cells were found in lymphoid organs of adult animals. Radiochemical analysis of lymphoid organs could only be carried out in 3-week-old and adult hamsters. It was found that significant migration of thymic cells occurred to mesenteric lymph nodes, Peyer's patches and spleen; in the 3-week-old group, significant transport of lymphoid cells to the spleen was observed only in male animals which may be of significance in view of the sex-linked occurrence of wasting in male hamsters (SHERMAN et al., 1963). Of particular importance is the demonstration of cell migration from the thymus to Peyer's patches in the guinea pig (LINNA and STILLSTRÖM, 1966) and to the tonsils in rabbits (LINNA, 1967 a) with regard to the hypothesis that these gut-associated lymphoid structures may be part of the mammalian "bursa equivalent" (see COOPER et al., 1967).

According to PARROT et al. (1966) and DeSousa and PARROT (1967), thymus-derived lymphoid cells preferentially localize in so-called "thymus-dependent areas" of mouse lymphoid tissue. When thymic lymphocytes were *in vitro* labeled with ^{3}H-adenosine and transfused into syngeneic recipients, surviving cells were found exclusively in the inner zone of the lymph node cortex and in a zone immediately adjacent to central arterioles of the spleen; in contrast, labeled spleen cells were found to be distributed evenly not only in the "thymus-dependent areas" but also in the outer cortex of lymph nodes and in peripheral follicles of the spleen. Lymphocyte depletion following neonatal thymectomy in mice appeared to be most marked in these "thymus-dependent areas". However, LEUCHARS et al. (1966) were able to demonstrate dividing thymic cells in lymphoid follicles of adult thymectomized and irradiated mice which carried a thymus graft of a mouse strain with a marker chromosome and, as pointed out by GOOD (1967), "thymus-dependent areas" in lymph nodes may not be identical in all animal species.

The main objection to the concept of "thymus-dependent areas" in lymph nodes is that it may be hazardous to relate the differential localization in lymph nodes of inoculated labeled cells from thymus, spleen and bone marrow to the behavior of these cells in the intact animal. The fact that transfused cells of different lymphoid organs may be found in different areas of lymph nodes may merely reflect differences in migratory capacities of these cells.

4. The Effects of Thymectomy on Antibody Formation

4.1. Neonatally Thymectomized Animals

In 1961, ARCHER and PIERCE reported on severe impairment of antibody-forming capacity in rabbits, thymectomized at the age of 5 to 7 days and stimulated 5 to 8 weeks later by a single intravenous injection of bovine serum albumin (BSA). During 3 weeks following antigenic stimulation, no precipitating antibodies against BSA could be detected in the serum of a total of 7 thymectomized rabbits while 9 out of 11 sham- or nonoperated control animals exhibited normal precipitin responses. It was concluded that the thymus was necessary for the normal development of antibody-forming tissue in rabbits.

This was the first in a series of enthusiastic reports which appeared during the following years on total or near-total abolition of antibody production after neonatal thymectomy. Soon it became clear, however, that the effects of neonatal thymectomy on humoral antibody formation vary from animal to animal, and from antigen to antigen; normal or only slightly depressed antibody responses following neonatal thymectomy were observed in rabbits (ARCHER et al., 1962), in mice (HESS et al., 1963, HUMPHREY et al., 1964; FAHEY et al., 1965; BASCH, 1966), and in rats (PINNAS and FITCH, 1966). In addition, and of great importance, several reports indicated that results depended to a large extent on whether the animals used were raised in a conventional or a specific pathogen-free or germfree environment (HESS et al., 1963; BEALMEAR and WILSON, 1967 a, b; McINTIRE et al., 1964). Accordingly, results obtained in conventional and specific pathogen-free or germfree animals will be treated separately in the following review.

4.1.1. Conventionally Raised Animals

4.1.1.1. Mice

Antibody production following neonatal thymectomy has been studied most extensively in mice (Table 3).

Studies on immunoglobulin production and turnover in thymectomized mice indicated that all immunoglobulins detectable in the serum of normal mice may be found in the serum of animals thymectomized at birth; the latter, however, were found to take longer to recover from physiological hypogammaglobulinemia of early life (HUMPHREY et al., 1964; ARNASON et al., 1964 a). No molecular abnormalities of the immunoglobulins could be detected (FAHEY et al., 1965). Levels of different types of immunoglobulins were found to be either increased or subnormal (HUMPHREY et al., 1964; ARNASON et al., 1964 a; FAHEY et al., 1965). Whether these reported differences are due to the different state of health of the mouse strains used or whether they merely reflect unresolved problems of immunoglobulin-terminology in mice is not clear. Increased rates of both synthesis *and* catabolism of IgG were observed predominantly in wasting animals, indicating perhaps an increased disappearance rate of antibody due to infectious processes.

Sheep red cells (SRC) were most widely used as antigenic material, and anti-SRC formation by neonatally thymectomized mice was reported to be

Table 3. *Humoral antibody formation in neonatally thymectomized conventional mice*

Antigen	Mouse strain	Wasting	Result	Authors
Sheep red cells	(Ak×T6)F$_1$	yes	Primary and secondary hemagglutinin responses impaired	MILLER, 1963
	C3H/Bi and (C57BL×C3H)F$_1$	yes	Variably impaired hemagglutinin responses	HUMPHREY et al., 1964
	C57BL/6 and ASn	?	No detectable hemagglutinin response; hemolysin formation impaired	SVET-MOLDAVSKY et al., 1964; ZINZAR and SVET-MOLDAVSKY, 1967
	A-Swiss	yes	Primary responses impaired, secondary responses not affected	ROGISTER, 1965
	Swiss and CBA	?	Hemagglutinin and hemolysin responses impaired	SINCLAIR, 1967
	C3Hf/Lw	yes	Hemagglutinin and hemolysin responses impaired	FAHEY et al., 1964
	LAF$_1$	yes	Primary hemolysin responses impaired; slight impairment also in shamoperated controls	SCHOOLEY et al., 1965
	C57BL	-yes	No detectable primary and secondary hemagglutinin responses	BASCH, 1966
	C57BL/6J	(yes)	No impairment of hemagglutinin responses	BROOKE, 1965
	Swiss (Tif 1)	no	Impairment of hemagglutinin and hemolysin responses only up to 3 months of age	DUKOR et al., 1966

Table 3 (continued)

Antigen	Mouse strain	Wasting	Result	Authors
Sheep red cells	(CBA×CBA-T6T6)F$_1$	yes	Impairment of hemagglutinin and hemolysin responses	Dukor et al., 1966
	NIH-Albino	yes	Impairment of hemolysin-plaque formation	Friedman, 1965
	CBA, SWS, and (Ak×T6)F$_1$	yes		Miller et al., 1965
	CF$_1$ and SL	?		Takeya et al., 1964
	(CBA×CBA-T6T6)F$_1$	yes		Dukor et al., 1966
	Swiss (Tif 1)	no	Impairment of hemolysin-plaque formation only up to 3 months	Dukor et al., 1966
Ovalbumin	Balb/c	no [a]	Impairment of precipitin formation	Arnason et al., 1964 a
Bovine serum albumine	Balb/c	no [a]	Impairment of precipitin formation	Arnason et al., 1964 a
	C57BL	yes		Basch, 1966
	C57BL/6J	(yes)		Brooke, 1965
Ferritin	C3Hf/Lw	yes	No impairment	Fahey et al., 1964
Hemocyanin	C3Hf/Lw	yes	Slight impairment	Fahey et al., 1964
	C3H/Bi and (C57BL×C3H)F$_1$	yes	No impairment	Humphrey et al., 1964
Salmonella typhi O-antigen	Balb/c	no [a]	No impairment of agglutinin formation	Arnason et al., 1964 a
	C3H/Bi and (C57BL×C3H)F$_1$	yes	Variable impairment of agglutinin formation	Humphrey et al., 1964
	C57BL/6 and ASn	yes	Primary agglutinin formation impaired; secondary response not affected	Zinzar and Svet-Moldavsky, 1967
H-antigen	(Ak×T6)F$_1$	yes	Severe impairment of agglutinin formation	Miller, 1963
	C3H/Bi and (C57BL×C3H)F$_1$	yes	Variable impairment of agglutinin formation	Humphrey et al., 1964

Table 3 (continued)

Antigen	Mouse strain	Wasting	Result	Authors
Vi-antigen	C57BL/6 and ASn	?	Slight to severe impairment	Svet-Moldavsky et al., 1964
S. typhimurium H-antigen	C57BL/6J	(yes)	No impairment of agglutinin formation	Brooke, 1965
Diphtheria toxoid	Balb/c	no [a]	Impairment of antitoxin formation	Arnason et al., 1964 a
Pneumococcus capsular polysaccharide	C3H/Bi and (C57BL×C3H)F$_1$	yes	No impairment	Humphrey et al., 1964
	C57BL/6J	(yes)	No impairment	Brooke, 1965
Coliphage T2	DBA/2	?	Marked impairment of neutralizing antibody formation	Good et al., 1962
M-S	C57BL	yes	No impairment of primary, but severe impairment of secondary antibody formation	Basch, 1966
Influenza A virus	(Ak×T6)F$_1$	yes	Severe impairment of agglutinin formation	Miller, 1963
Influenza ? virus	C57BL/6 and ASn	?	Slight to severe impairment of agglutinin formation	Svet-Moldavsky et al., 1964
Polyoma virus	C3H/Bi	yes	Impairment of agglutinin formation	Defendi et al., 1964
	C3Hf/HeN and (C57BL×C3H)F$_1$	yes [b]	Impairment of agglutinin formation	Ting and Law, 1965

[a] Thymectomy at 4 days of age.

[b] No wasting and no impairment of antibody formation when thymectomized at 3 days of age.

severely depressed in most cases. Failure to produce anti-SRC hemagglutinins in response to primary and secondary stimulation in 4 to 6-week-old neonatally thymectomized (Ak×T6)F_1 mice was noted by MILLER (1963). HUMPHREY et al. (1964) usually, but not always, found depressed antibody responses in C3H/Bi and (C57BL×C3H/Bi)F_1 mice; it should be noted that these authors administered a mixture of SRC, hemocyanin and pneumococcus type III polysaccharide by simultaneous intravenous injection. Neonatal thymectomy completely abolished the ability of C57BL/6 and Sn mice to form anti-SRC hemagglutinins at 1 to 2 months after the operation, whereas hemolysins were always measurable, though variably depressed; normal hemagglutinin formation was observed after repeated antigen administration (SVET-MOLDAVSKY et al., 1964; ZINZAR and SVET-MOLDAVSKY, 1967). Similar findings were reported by ROGISTER (1964) in A-Sw mice and by SINCLAIR (1967) in outbred Swiss and CBA mice. Markedly impaired hemolysin and agglutinin responses were obtained in C3Hf/Lw mice 1 and 2 weeks after stimulation (FAHEY et al., 1965). A depression of primary hemolysin responses in both neonatally thymectomized and, to a lesser degree, in sham-operated LAF$_1$ mice was reported by SCHOOLEY et al. (1965). In contrast, BASCH (1966) could detect neither primary nor secondary hemagglutinin responses in C57BL mice which had been stimulated by the injection of either 0.6 or 0.06 mg of SRC-stromata in all 4 footpads 3 weeks after neonatal thymectomy. Hemolysin and hemagglutinin responses were depressed in neonatally thymectomized Swiss albino mice (Tif 1 strain) when the animals were stimulated before the age of 9 to 13 weeks; 3-month-old thymectomized mice had titers identical to those of controls. A similar "recovery" of immunologic responsiveness after neonatal thymectomy was not observed in (CBA×CBA-T6T6)F_1 mice which, in contrast to the Swiss mice, showed a marked incidence of wasting disease (DUKOR et al., 1966).

In an attempt to clarify whether the observed depressive effect of neonatal thymectomy on antibody production after stimulation with SRC was due to a qualitative defect of antibody-producing cells or to a quantitative deficiency in the number of responding cells, use was made of the JERNE plaque technique for the enumeration of hemolysin-producing spleen cells (JERNE et al., 1963). Independent studies carried out by FRIEDMAN (1965) on NIH albino mice, by MILLER et al. (1965) on CBA, (T6×Ak)F_1 and Swiss mice, and by TAKEYA et al. on CF$_1$ and inbred SL mice (TAKEYA et al., 1964; TAKEYA and NOMOTO, 1967), yielded closely similar results: the number of plaque-forming cells found in the spleens of thymectomized animals was distinctly lower than that found in spleens of sham- or nonoperated controls; the amount of hemolysin produced by single cells (as judged by the size of single plaques) appeared to be identical in all groups. The general conclusion was that in response to SRC very few or no hemolysin-plaque forming cells were produced in the spleens of neonatally thymectomized animals, but that the antibody-forming capacity of single spleen cells was not impaired in the absence of the thymus.

Serumproteins, such as ovalbumin or bovine serum albumin (BSA), proved to be "weak" antigens in neonatally thymectomized mice. Severe impairment of precipitin formation following stimulation with ovalbumin and BSA was observed in Balb/c mice, thymectomized at 4 days of age (ARNASON et al., 1964 a). BASCH (1966) found no appreciable primary or secondary anti-BSA production in neonatally thymectomized C57BL mice following stimulation with BSA in saline in all footpads. Antigenic stimulation with highmolecular weight proteins, such as hemocyanin and ferritin, was followed by normal or near-normal antibody formation, even in wasting neonatally thymectomized C3H/Lw (FAHEY et al., 1965), C3H/Bi and (C57BL×C3H/Bi)F$_1$ mice (HUMPHREY et al., 1964).

Antibody responses to bacteria or bacterial products were variably affected by neonatal thymectomy. Following intraperitoneal stimulation with *Salmonella typhi* O- and H-antigen, agglutinin responses of neonatally thymectomized C3H/Bi and (C57BL×C3H/Bi)F$_1$ mice were usually, but not always, depressed (HUMPHREY et al., 1964). MILLER (1963) reported that from 50 to 80⁰/₀ of thymectomized (Ak×T6)F$_1$ mice failed to produce antibodies to *S. typhi* H-antigen. On the other hand, neonatally thymectomized C57BL/6 and Sn mice were able to respond to stimulation with *S. typhi* Vi-antigen although titers were lower than in nonoperated controls (SVET-MOLDAVSKY et al., 1964); animals of the same mouse strains had impaired primary responses to *S. typhi* O-antigen while secondary responses were normal (ZINZAR and SVET-MOLDAVSKY, 1967). Normal responses to *S. typhimurium* H-antigen could be elicited in C57BL/6J mice which had been stimulated 9 weeks after neonatal thymectomy; wasting was reported to be "negligible" (BROOKE, 1965). It appears noteworthy that normal responses to *S. typhi* O-antigen were observed only in a strain of conventional mice which did not exhibit signs of postthymectomy wasting (ARNASON et al., 1964 a); this finding was interpreted by these authors to mean that antibodies belonging to the IgM class of immunoglobulins could be produced normally in thymectomized animals while the formation of antibodies belonging to the IgA and IgG classes was much more affected in the absence of the thymus. More than 50⁰/₀ of neonatally thymectomized C3H/Bi and (C57BL×C3H/Bi)F$_1$ mice responded as well as or better than nonoperated controls to stimulation with an immunizing dose of type III pneumococcus capsular polysaccharide (HUMPHREY et al., 1964). Diphtheria antitoxin formation was severely impaired in thymectomized Balb/c mice (ARNASON et al., 1964 a).

Antibody formation following stimulation with viral antigens was not always impaired following neonatal thymectomy. PAPERMASTER et al. (1962 b) and GOOD et al. (1962) found a drastically impaired ability of

60-day-old neonatally thymectomized DBA/2 mice to produce neutralizing antibody against T2 coliphage. In contrast, normal primary antibody responses following stimulation with M-S coliphage were observed in thymectomized C57BL mice (BASCH, 1966). While MILLER (1963) reported on the failure of from 50 to 80% of thymectomized (Ak$\times$T6)F$_1$ mice to produce measurable amounts of agglutinating antibody to influenza A virus, depressed but demonstrable hemagglutination-inhibiting antibody was observed in thymectomized C57BL/6 and Sn mice following stimulation with influenza virus (SVET-MOLDAVSKY et al., 1964). DEFENDI et al. (1964) and TING and LAW (1965) observed the production of significant levels of antiviral antibody in neonatally thymectomized C3H and (C3H$\times$C57BL)F$_1$ mice which had been infected with polyoma virus.

4.1.1.2. Species other than Mice

The effects of neonatal thymectomy on antibody formation in animal species other than mice have been studied with a small spectrum of antigens only. A synopsis of experimental results is presented in Table 4.

JANKOVIC et al. (1962) and ARNASON et al. (1964 b) noted failure of neonatally thymectomized Sprague-Dawley rats to produce significant titers of precipitating and hemagglutinating antibody following stimulation with BSA in complete Freund's adjuvant. Eight-week-old neonatally thymectomized Lewis rats were unable to produce precipitating antibody, and only 6 out of 17 animals produced hemagglutinating antibody at 15 days after stimulation with BSA (ISAKOVIC et al., 1965 a). The impairment of precipitin-formation following stimulation with horse serum proteins could be reduced by maintaining the animals on antibiotics, reducing at the same time the incidence of wasting disease (AZAR et al., 1964). ARNASON et al. (1964 c) reported on impaired antibody formation in neonatally thymectomized WAG (Wistar) rats following stimulation with diphtheria toxoid and BSA while responses to *Salmonella typhi* O-antigen and pneumococcus type 2 were only insignificantly depressed; defective antibody formation was correlated to the reduced capacity of neonatally thymectomized rats to produce significant levels of IgA immunoglobulins. In a more recent study, PINNAS and FITCH (1966) noted that neonatally thymectomized CFN rats were unable to form measurable anti-BSA antibody when stimulated at 4 weeks of age; however, stimulation at 10 or 16 weeks was followed by formation of both hemagglutinating and precipitating antibodies, although titers of thymectomized animals remained lower than those measured in nonoperated controls. Neonatal thymectomy had no depressing effect on agglutinin titers after stimulation with SRC, or stimulation with particular and soluble flagellar antigen of *S. typhi;* the number of hemolysin plaque forming cells in the spleens of these animals was not depressed by neonatal thymectomy.

Table 4. *Humoral antibody formation in neonatally thymectomized conventional animals others than mice*

Species and strain	Antigen	Result	Authors
Rat Sprague-Dawley	BSA	Impairment (precipitin and passive hemagglutination)	JANKOVIC et al., 1962 ARNASON et al., 1964 b
Lewis	Horse serum	Impaired precipitin formation	AZAR et al., 1964
CFN	BSA	No responses when stimulated at 4 weeks; impairment when stimulated at 10 or 16 weeks	PINNAS and FITCH, 1966
	Sheep Red Cells	No impairment of hemagglutinin or hemolysin-plaque formation	
	Salmonella typhi flagellar antigen	No impairment	
WAG (Wistar)	Diphtheria toxoid	Impaired antitoxin formation	ARNASON et al., 1964 c
	BSA	Impaired precipitin formation	
	S. typhi O Pneumococcus	No impairment	
Rabbit New Zealand	BSA BGG	Slight to severe impairment, especially when thymectomy combined with appendectomy	GOOD et al., 1962 ARCHER et al., 1964 a
	T2-coliphage	Slight impairment	SHERMAN et al., 1964
Hamster	HGG	Impairment when operated within 2 weeks after birth	DEFENDI et al., 1964
	Polyoma virus	Slight impairment	

In rabbits, neonatal thymectomy, especially when combined with appendectomy, was severely impairing antibody formation against BSA and bovine gammaglobulin (BGG) (GOOD et al., 1962; ARCHER et al., 1964 a, b). On the other hand, the same strain of rabbits (New Zealand albino) showed only minimal impairment of antibody formation against T2-coliphage when thymectomized at birth, and responses to BSA were only slightly lower than those of controls when thymectomy was performed at the age of 5 to 7 days.

In neonatally thymectomized Syrian hamsters *(Mesocricetus aureus)*, antibody responses were severely depressed following stimulation with human gammaglobulin (HGG) (SHERMAN et al., 1964) whereas only slight impairment of formation of polyoma virus agglutinin was reported (DEFENDI et al., 1964). It should be noted that wasting was observed in hamsters as an unexplained sex-linked occurrence (SHERMAN et al., 1963; ADNER et al., 1955), a phenomenon which has not been confirmed by other investigators (ROOSA et al., 1965).

4.2.1. Specific Pathogen-free and Germfree Animals

In a series of studies, the effects of neonatal thymectomy on tetanus antitoxin formation were tested in specific pathogen-free albino mice (BNL-Swiss, Hale-Stoner strain). In a first experiment (HESS et al., 1963) a total of 68 mice was thymectomized within 24 hours after birth, or at 1, 4 or 8 days of age. All mice were given a primary injection of aluminum phosphate absorbed tetanus toxoid (APTT) at the age of 4 weeks. Three weeks later blood was collected by tail-artery bleeding for titration of antitoxin produced during the primary response. Later in the same day, all animals were given a booster injection of fluid tetanus toxoid (FTT) to elicit secondary responses. The animals were sacrificed for serum 10 days after the second antigenic stimulus.

As evident from Fig. 5, antitoxin titers of one-third of all thymectomized animals were lower than the lowest titer found in non-operated controls. Antitoxin levels varied considerably in thymectomized mice while titers of nonoperated controls were more uniform. The ability of thymectomized mice to respond to secondary antigenic stimulation was impaired to a greater extent than the capacity to respond to primary injection. In two-thirds of thymectomized animals, antitoxin titers were repressed below the lowest titer measured in control mice. In contrast to the more varied results observed with primary responses, secondary antitoxin formation was more uniformly depressed in animals thymectomized on day 1 through day 8. When antitoxin titers of thymectomized animals were compared to those of their respective littermate controls by the Wilcoxon test, it was found that whereas primary responses of thymectomized animals were not always significantly repressed, secondary responses in all groups as a whole were significantly lower than titers measured in the respective control groups. While post-thymectomy wasting was not observed among operated animals, no correlation could be found between the amount of antitoxin produced after primary and secondary stimulation. Several thymectomized animals with fairly good primary responses produced minimal amounts of antitoxin after secondary stimulation; several animals with low primary responses, on the other hand, showed excellent secondary responses.

The same overall response pattern of neonatally thymectomized BNL-Swiss mice was observed when primary stimulation was given at the age of

either 4, 7, 10, or 15 weeks, and secondary responses were elicited in all
animals at the age of 20 weeks: while primary antitoxin responses were
moderately impaired, secondary antitoxin production was drastically re-

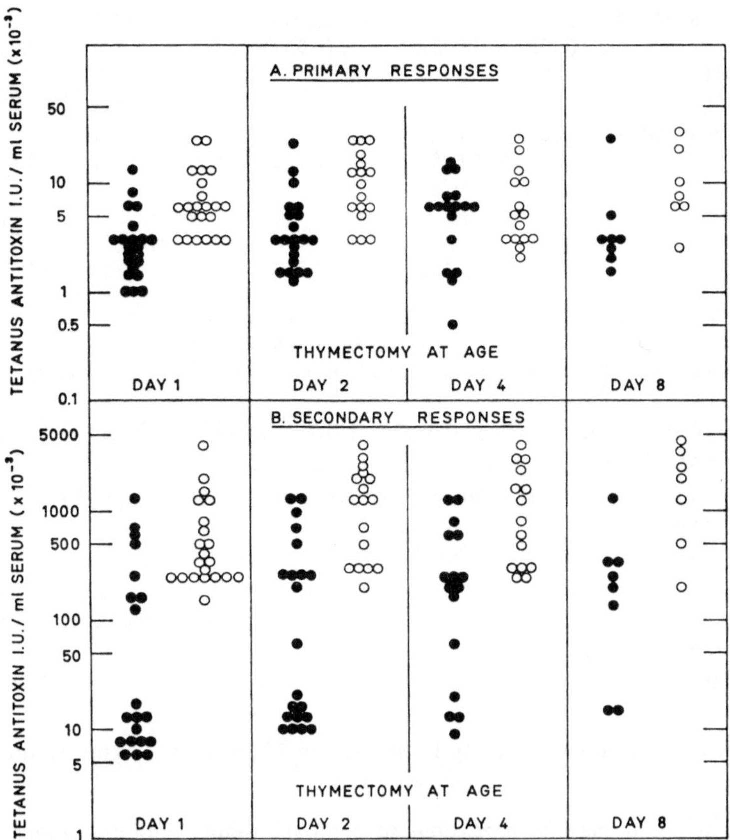

Fig. 5. Primary and secondary tetanus antitoxin responses in BNL-Swiss mice
thymectomized at various time intervals after birth (closed circles: thymectomized
animals; open circles: nonoperated littermate controls)

pressed or absent in a group of animals (Fig. 6). In the animals only feebly
reacting to second antigenic stimulation, a complete refractoriness to a third
antigenic stimulus was observed (Table 5) (HESS and STONER, 1966).

Stimulation of neonatally thymectomized BNL-Swiss mice with per-
tussis vaccine resulted in agglutinin titers not different from those elicited in
sham- or nonoperated controls; likewise, no significant depressive effect of
neonatal thymectomy could be detected on responses of 26-week-old mice
to stimulation with heat-aggregated BSA (HESS and STONER, 1967 b).

Table 5. *Tetanus antitoxin responses after third antigenic stimulation*

Experimental condition	Mean titers expressed as I.U. antitoxin/ml serum					
	N	Primary [a]	N	Secondary [b]	N	Tertiary [c]
Thymectomized (impaired secondary responses)	16	0.0016 (0.0009—0.0025)	16	0.0214 (0.0063—0.055)	13 / 3	0.010 (0.005—0.0625) / 1.9 (0.875—3.625)
Thymectomized (normal secondary responses)	13	0.0038 (0.0009—0.0250)	13	3.0 (0.250—7.00)	13	9.0 (1.375—12.5)
Nonoperated littermates	16	0.0040 (0.0009—0.0250)	16	3.5 (0.250—6.25)	16	7.5 (0.45—12.5)

[a] 3 weeks after 0.05 ml APTT s.c. (injected at age 4 to 16 weeks)
[b] 10 days after 0.10 ml FTT s.c. (injected at age 20 weeks)
[c] 6 days after 0.05 ml FTT in each hind foot pad (injected at age 30 weeks)

Thymectomy during the first week of life in specific pathogen-free Long-Evans rats did not affect the ability of these animals to respond to either primary or secondary stimulation with *Salmonella adelaide* (SCHOOLEY and KELLY, 1964).

Limited information is available at the present time on antibody formation in neonatally thymectomized germfree animals. Stimulation with *Salmonella typhimurium* H-antigen of neonatally thymectomized germfree CBA and C57BL mice resulted in agglutinin titers equal to or higher than those elicited in nonoperated controls (BEALMEAR and WILSON, 1967 b).

4.1.3. Discussion of Antibody Formation in Neonatally Thymectomized Animals

Although it may be hazardous to compare results obtained under such dissimilar experimental approaches, it appears to emerge quite distinctly that thymectomy effects vary with
1) the general health of the animals,
2) kind and physical form of antigen used,
3) the age of the animals at the time of stimulation,
4) the method used for antibody measurement, and
5) whether or not a clear distinction was made between primary and secondary antigenic stimulation.

The phenomenon of *"post-thymectomy wasting"* will be discussed in some detail in a later section. However, it seems quite clear that, under certain conditions, the process of wasting may grossly distort the evaluation of the effects of neonatal thymectomy on antibody formation. Whereas most observations on the impairment of antibody formation were obtained in conventionally raised animals, it should be emphasized that normal or near-normal responses to a number of antigens have been regularly obtained in neonatally thymectomized, specific-pathogen-free (HESS et al., 1963; HESS and STONER, 1966; SCHOOLEY and KELLY, 1964) or germfree animals (BEALMEAR and WILSON, 1967 b) in which wasting does not occur. AZAR (1964) reported that by maintaining neonatally thymectomized rats on an antibiotic (tetracycline) not only was the incidence of wasting reduced but also an improvement of the capacity to form precipitating antibodies to horse proteins was noted as compared to nontreated thymectomized control animals. In a direct comparison, BEALMEAR and WILSON (1967 b) tested the ability of conventionally raised and germfree mice of the same strain to respond to primary stimulation with *Salmonella typhimurium* following neonatal thymectomy; responses of conventionally raised mice were severely impaired while germfree animals had titers similar to or better than those obtained in nonoperated controls. In addition, it was reported that neonatally thymectomized C3H and (C57BL×C3H)F_1 mice eventually died from wasting disease and exhibited impaired formation of hemagglutination-inhibiting antibody against polyoma virus while animals of the same strain did not develop wasting and responded normally to stimulation with polyoma virus when thymectomized at 3 days of age (LAW et al., 1964). This particular observation was explained on the basis of the hypothesis that wasting and defective antibody-forming mechanisms may in part be independent effects of thymectomy.

One gains the impression that, particularly in animals strains which are susceptible to wasting, *choice of the antigen* significantly affects the outcome of the experiments. Responses to "good" antigens, such as hemocyanin, ferritin, coliphage, pneumococcus polysaccharide and tetanus toxoid, appear to be more difficult to suppress by neonatal thymectomy than responses to "weak" antigens, such as serum proteins or diphtheria toxoid (in mice).

Responses to BSA were reported to be depressed in neonatally thymectomized animals when the antigen was incorporated into Freund's adjuvant (ARNASON et al., 1964 a; BROOKE, 1965) or when administered in a saline solution (BASCH, 1966); in a limited number of thymectomized, specific pathogen-free BNL-Swiss mice, responses to stimulation with heat-denatured BSA were only slightly impaired (HESS and STONER, 1967 b). In other systems, however, the physical nature and relative antigenicity of the antigen do not appear to be decisive factors. Neonatally thymectomized BNL-Swiss mice responded equally well to tetanus toxoid in a fluid form, absorbed to aluminum phosphate, or in complex with isologous antitoxin at equivalence, although titers were slightly lower than those of controls (HESS and STONER, 1966; HESS and STONER, 1967 a). PINNAS and FITCH (1966) found identical responses of thymectomized CFN rats following stimulation with *Salmonella typhi* flagellar antigen, administered either in particulate or in soluble form. The antigenic dose may also play a role, especially if the induction of immunosuppression (tolerance or paralysis) depends on a critical ratio of antigenic dose to the number of cells. Since thymectomized animals have a reduced number of immunologically competent cells, it is proposed that humoral antibody responses are suppressed by antigenic doses which, in normal animals, induce antibody formation (HUMPHREY et al., 1964; BROOKE, 1965; HESS and STONER, 1967 a). The finding of normal antibody formation in thymectomized mice following the injection of immunizing doses of pneumococcus polysaccharide (HUMPHREY et al., 1964; BROOKE, 1965), a substance with which the induction of paralysis of antibody formation depends critically on the administered dose (FELTON et al., 1955), makes this explanation unlikely. It may be mentioned also that it was impossible to induce immunological tolerance in neonatally thymectomized Swiss mice by the perinatal injection of large doses of tetanus toxoid in various physical forms (HESS and STONER, 1967 a, b).

The role which the *age at immunization* may play in affecting antibody formation by neonatal thymectomy has been studied in pathogen-free BNL-Swiss mice (HESS and STONER, 1966). A total of 129 mice were thymectomized either immediately after birth or at the age of 2 to 4 days; comparable numbers of sham-or nonoperated littermates served as controls. Primary antitoxin responses of both groups of thymectomized and sham-operated animals, stimulated at the age of 4, 7, 10, or 15 weeks, are presented in Fig. 6. Titers of all groups were higher when the primary antigenic stimulation was given at 15 weeks of age as compared to responses obtained following stimulation at the age of 4 weeks. Titers of thymectomized animals remained slightly below those obtained in the control groups (significant difference revealed by Wilcoxon tests). It was concluded that extension of time intervals between thymectomy and primary stimulation up to 15 weeks had no influence on the depressive effect of the operation. This finding does not readily fit the hypothesis that the reduced number of immunologically active cells in thymectomized animals may become "committed" in early postnatal life to antibody production against environmental antigens thus reducing the number of "noncommitted" cells capable to react with newly encountered antigens in later life (ARNASON et al., 1964 a; LAW, 1966; GOOD, 1967). PINNAS and FITCH (1966) found that neonatally thymectomized rats were unable to respond to foot-pad stimulation with BSA in complete Freund's adjuvant when the antigen was injected at the age of 4 weeks, although responses to other antigens (SRC, flagellar *Salmonella typhi* antigens) could be elicited at that age. Antibody formation to BSA was present following stimulation at 10 weeks and had further improved at 16 weeks of age, although titers of thymectomized rats remained below titers elicited in sham- or nonoperated controls. These results were

interpreted as further evidence for the hypothesis, originally proposed by
SILVERSTEIN (1962), that the acquisition of competence to various antigens
may be a stepwise process during fetal and neonatal life. It was concluded
that the competence of rats to react with antibody formation following

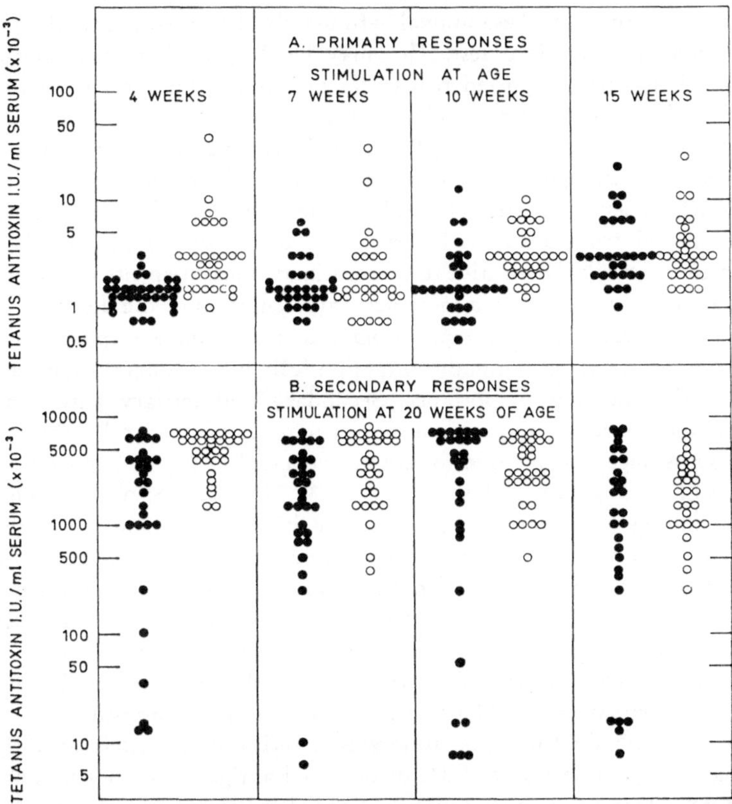

Fig. 6. Primary and secondary tetanus antitoxin responses in neonatally thymectomized BNL-Swiss mice; time intervals between operation and primary stimulation
varied (closed circles: thymectomized animals; open circles: shamoperated controls)

stimulation with BSA was acquired only after birth. BASCH (1966), on the
basis of the same hypothesis, argued that deprivation of an animal by
thymectomy of one or more thymic factors required to initiate and maintain
the proliferation of immunologically competent cells before the appearance
of an adequate number of cells capable to respond to antigenic stimulation
would prevent the manifestation of competence for that antigen. PINNAS
and FITCH (1966), however, demonstrated, under the conditions of their
experiment, that the development of competence occurred even in the
absence of the thymus.

The availability of sensitive *methods for antibody determination* may be of great importance, especially when working with antigens against which even control animals produce only little antibody. It may be fallacious to conclude abolition of antibody-forming capacities in thymectomized animals on the basis of nondetectable antibody; more sensitive methods may reveal that antibody titers in these animals are merely depressed below the sensitivity level of a standard test. This may be illustrated by the following example: it has been reported repeatedly that bursectomized chickens were unable to form humoral antibody against a series of antigens (see section 4.3); however, CLAFLIN et al. (1966), by increasing the sensitivity of an agglutination technique, could demonstrate normal amounts of mercapto-ethanol (ME)-sensitive (IgM?) antibody in bursaless chickens following intraperitoneal stimulation with *Brucella abortus* organismus. Maybe the application of similarly sensitive tests to antibody measurements in thymecto-mized animals could lead to a more accurate definition of the defect.

The *distinction between true primary and secondary responses* in the evaluation of defects in antibody formation following neonatal thymectomy may be of paramount importance. Secondary and tertiary antitoxin responses were more severely impaired in a number of neonatally thymecto-mized Swiss mice as compared to responses elicited in sham- or nonoperated controls (Figs. 5 and 6) (HESS et al., 1963; HESS and STONER, 1966). A similar finding has been reported recently by BASCH (1966). Neonatally thymectomized C57BL mice were stimulated with various doses of MS-2 coliphage either immediately after the operation or at 5 to 6 weeks of age. All animals produced phage-neutralizing antibody following primary stimu-lation. Secondary responses elicited 25 days after primary injection were markedly reduced and delayed in pratically all thymectomized mice.

In this context it should be emphasized that it is impossible to study "primary" antibody formation following a series of injections of antigen, and that a single injection of SRC or bacterial antigens does not necessarily constitute a true primary stimulation since there may exist a more or less continuous stimulation with crossreacting antigens from gut-associated organisms or from latent infections. It is of interest to note that, although no impairment of primary and secondary responses to *Salmonella typhi* flagellar antigen was reported in thymectomized rats, neither experimental nor control animals exhibited impressive titer increases following secondary stimulation (PINNAS and FITCH, 1966). Similarly, there is no striking differ-ence between primary and secondary titers elicited by stimulation with SRC. This lack of titer increases following secondary stimulation with a number of antigens may indicate that responses elicited with these antigens are always "anamnestic".

The finding that neonatal thymectomy in a group of animals has more severe effects on secondary than on primary antibody formation following stimulation with some antigens was not anticipated. Possible explanations for this phenomenon have been presented, in part, by HESS et al. (1963), BASCH (1966), and HESS and STONER (1966).

1. The possibility was considered earlier that immunologically competent cells might have left the thymus before the operation and reached the end of their lifespan prior to secondary stimulation; the lifespan of these peripheralized and sensitized cells may thus be the limiting factor in the absence of the thymus (HESS et al., 1963). A similar view was expressed by DE VRIES et al. (1962) who concluded from morphological studies that thymectomy was followed by progressive self-destruction of the lymphoid cell population. However, since similar depressions of primary antitoxin responses were obtained in mice stimulated as late as 15 weeks after neonatal thymectomy, and since, in addition, depression of secondary responses was observed to be more pronounced in some animals of all groups, it may not be assumed that an altered lifespan of antibody-forming cells alone could account for the observed phenomenon (HESS and STONER, 1966).

2. By removal of the thymus in the neonatal animal, the organism is depleted of a large fraction of its lymphoid cell population. This may cause a sharp reduction in the number of cells available to react to primary antigenic stimulation with proliferation and/or maturation to antibody-forming cells. Since it has been shown that there are few cell divisions among lymphoid cells during primary responses (ALBRIGHT and MAKINODAN, 1965) as compared to the explosive proliferation noted during secondary responses (COTTIER et al., 1964 a, 1967), the number of cells capable of responding to secondary antigenic stimulation in thymectomized animals may be reduced below a critical level for successful completion of a secondary response.

Both hypotheses, however, offer no explanation for the fact that secondary responses may be severely depressed only in some animals. It cannot be excluded that scarring at the operation site may also be responsible, in part, for the observed effect; interference with lymphocyte recirculation by obstruction of the thoracic duct is likely to occur.

4.2. Animals Thymectomized in Adult Life

HAMMAR (1938) was the first to study the influence of the thymus on immune reactivity in adult rabbits. The animals were thymectomized and immunized with a series of weekly injections of *Salmonella paratyphi B* organisms, starting 8 weeks after the operation. Formation of anti-H agglutinin was slightly impaired in thymectomized animals as compared to non-operated controls; the difference in the observed titers was not statistically significant. In similar experiments performed with rabbits, thymectomized in adult life, HARRIS et al. (1948) and MACLEAN et al. (1957) observed no impairment of antibody formation against *Shigella paradysenteriae, Salmonella typhi,* SRC or BSA. FICHTELIUS et al. (1961) studied primary and secondary responses of partially thymectomized adult guinea pigs to immunization with *Salmonella typhi* H-antigen. Agglutinin titers at 7 days after primary stimulation were lower in thymectomized as compared to shamoperated animals; no difference in titers of operated and shamoperated guinea pigs was observed at 7 days after secondary antigenic stimulation. C3H/HeJ mice, thymectomized at the age of 3 months, responded as well as controls to multiple injections of human gammaglobulin despite drastically reduced levels of circulating lymphocytes (AZAR et al., 1963).

These results have led to the conclusion that "the thymus gland (in young rabbits) does not participate in the control of the immune response" (MACLEAN et al., 1957). However, renewed efforts towards elucidating thymic function in the adult organism produced results which cast considerable doubt on this conclusion.

MILLER (1962 a) observed that $(Ak \times T6) F_1$ mice which were thymectomized at the age of 12 weeks and exposed to a single dose of 350 r wholebody X-radiation 2 weeks after the operation had not recovered their ability to produce SRC-agglutinins at 4 weeks after radiation exposure; shamoperated controls produced normal amounts of hemagglutinins within the same time interval after irradiation. Similar results were obtained by MILLER et al. (1963) and CROSS et al. (1962) in CBA mice in which thymectomy at the age of 9 to 10 weeks was combined with lethal wholebody irradiation. At one week after the operation, thymectomized and shamoperated animals were exposed to a single dose of 850 r X-radiation and protected by an intravenous injection of 5×10^6 homologous bone marrow cells. Thymectomized animals failed to produce hemagglutinins following either primary or secondary stimulation with SRC when tested from 4 to 10 weeks after irradiation; with these time intervals, both thymectomized, sham-irradiated and shamoperated, irradiated controls produced hemagglutinins. Thus, it has been demonstrated that, under these experimental conditions, the thymus may be necessary for complete recovery of immune mechanisms after radiation in adult life. Studies by BARNES et al. (1962), DAVIS et al. (1964), LEONARD and HUTCHINSON (1962), and TYAN and COLE (1967) confirmed these conclusions. However, DUKOR et al. (1966) found that Swiss albino mice (Tif 1 strain), thymectomized and irradiated at the age of 5 to 6 weeks, regained their ability to produce hemagglutinin and hemolysin responses following stimulation with SRC within 3 to 5 weeks after radiation; no recovery of hemolysin plaque forming capacity was noted.

While attempts to enhance the immunosuppressive action of Melphalan (L-phenylalanine mustard) by adult thymectomy failed (LUMB and SYMES, 1965), recent observations by DUKOR and DIETRICH (1967) suggest that cyclophosphamide-induced suppression of anti-SRC antibody formation may be potentiated by adult thymectomy in mice. Apparently, immuno-suppression by combined drug administration, radiation, and/or thymectomy depends critically on the particular compound used and/or the treatment schedule (GLOBERSON et al., 1962; DUKOR and DIETRICH, 1967).

While no immunological defects could be demonstrated in adult thymec-tomized and irradiated dogs (MCKNEALLY and OLIVERAS, 1965), responses of 3-week-old rabbits, thymectomized and/or appendectomized and exposed to 450 r X-radiation, to simultaneous immunization with *Salmonella typhi* and conalbumin were equivocal. Normal formation of anti-H-agglutinins with depressed responses to conalbumin were observed in animals following combined thymectomy and radiation; animals which were appendectomized and irradiated formed no *Salmonella* agglutinins and only reduced amounts of anti-conalbumin antibodies; following a combination of thymectomy, appendectomy and irradiation, depressed but measurable antibody forma-tion to both antigens was found. It should also be noted that non-irradiated control animals, including rabbits which were only thymectomized, only appendectomized or nonoperated, produced titers to both antigens which were identical to antibody responses elicited in nonoperated, irradiated controls (KONDA and HARRIS, 1966).

A study on immunoglobulin formation in adult thymectomized and irradiated mice, in general, revealed changes very similar to those observed in neonatally thymectomized animals: a slight, irregular diminution of IgG immunoglobulins together with an increase in IgA was noted by BAZIN and DUPLAN (1966). An infrequent but significant finding of these authors deserves further attention. Mice which were protected with adult spleen or bone marrow cells following a lethal dose of 850 r X-radiation developed normally and had normal immunoglobulin levels. However, if the protec-tive injection after lethal irradiation consisted of fetal liver cells (isologous fetus on 14th day of gestation) a marked diminution in the number of small lymphocytes in lymphoid organs together with the appearance of chronic wasting was noted. In two cases typical dysglobulinemias of the IgG_2 immunoglobulins developed, once in a mouse which had received a sublethal dose of 600 r, in the other case in a lethally irradiated mouse which had been injected with fetal liver cells. It is not known whether this "anarchic" production of gammaglobulin (BAZIN and DUPLAN, 1966) is due to the formation of a monoclonal, specific antibody or whether it indicates that gammaglobulin formation may be deranged in the absence of the thymus.

The marked depressive effect of combined thymectomy, irradiation and/or chemical immunotherapy on immune responsiveness may be due to slower and less complete regeneration of the lymphoid tissues after radiation (MILLER et al., 1963; FELDMAN and GLOBERSON, 1964; DUKOR and DIET-RICH, 1967). On the basis that defects similar to those observed after combined adult thymectomy and irradiation may become evident also after thymectomy alone, METCALF (1965, 1966 a) studied immune responses of mice, thymectomized at the age of 6 weeks and stimulated at intervals varying from one week to 18 months after the operation; C57BL and $(AKR \times C57BL)F_1$ mice were given a single intraperitoneal injection of SRC. Whereas no difference between hemagglutin titers of thymectomized and shamoperated mice was observed when the animals were stimulated shortly after the operation, titers elicited at 11 months after thymectomy were statistically lower in thymectomized as compared to titers elicited in control animals. When thymectomy preceded antigenic stimulation by 18 months, more than 50% of animals failed to produce detectable hemagglutinin titers; titers of the remaining half of thymectomized animals were found not to differ from the variable and low hemagglutinin responses observed normally in this age group. Similar delayed effects of adult thymectomy on immunological responsiveness to SRC and BSA were reported by MILLER (1965 a) and TAYLOR (1965). MILLER thymectomized 2- to 3-month-old CBA and $(Ak \times T6)F_1$ mice and stimulated with SRC at from 2 to 22 months after the operation; thymectomized animals had fewer hemolysin plaque forming cells in their spleens than nonoperated controls when 9 or more months elapsed between thymectomy and antigenic stimulation. In CBA mice, thymectomized at 4 or at 10 to 14 weeks of age, TAYLOR observed signs of an impaired capacity to respond to BSA already 10 to 16 weeks after the operation. However, JEEJEEBHOY (1965) reported that Sprague-Dawley rats, thymectomized at the age of 12 weeks, showed no decrease in their anti-SRC hemagglutinin or tetanus antitoxin production even when tested as late as 9 months after thymectomy. These latter findings are in agreement with results obtained in *neonatally* thymectomized animals in which stimulation with certain antigens as late as 16 to 25 weeks after the operation was not causing an impressive impairment of antibody responses (HESS and STONER, 1966, 1967 b; PINNAS and FITCH, 1966). Thus, it appears that in adult thymectomized animals the decline in the capacity to form antibodies against certain antigens occurs more rapidly than that observed with the use of other antigens.

4.3. Thymectomy and Acquired Immunological Tolerance

Mechanisms underlying the phenomenon of immunological tolerance are still unknown. According to current hypotheses tolerance may be the direct consequence of a reduction in the number of cells with the potential to form antibody against a given antigen, or of interference with effective induction of antibody formation (see BURNET, 1961; SMITH, 1961; EISEN and KARUSH, 1964). It has been shown recently by ROWLEY and FITCH (1965 a, b), using the hemolysin plaque-forming technique, that an animal which has been made tolerant to SRC has fewer plaque-forming cells in the spleen than nontolerant controls, and that no or only minimal proliferation of these cells occurs after a booster injection of the antigen. Persistence of antigen appears to be of importance in maintaining the tolerant state (CAMPBELL and GARVEY, 1963; ADA et al., 1965). A key role has been attributed to the thymus in the induction and maintenance of tolerance. It has been postulated by BURNET (1962) that the thymus acts as the main generator and/or modifier of lymphoid cells with the ability to react to antigenic stimulation, constantly eliminating cells with the potential to react with autologous, "self" components. On the basis of their studies on tolerance induction to flagellar proteins of *Salmonella adelaide*, NOSSAL and MITCHELL (1966) recently proposed that tolerance would ensue only when all lymphoid cells in the organism were exposed to the antigen in a non-phagocytized form, and in particular, when thymic lymphoid cells also came in contact with antigenic material.

Thymectomy of adult mice and rats, tolerant to bovine serum proteins, drastically delayed the reappearance of immune reactivity when antigen injections ceased (CLAMAN and TALMAGE, 1963; CLAMAN and MCDONALD, 1964). "Transfer of tolerance" to bovine gammaglobulin by transplanting thymic tissue from tolerant rats into thymectomized and irradiated non-tolerant recipients has been reported by ISAKOVIC et al. (1965). TOULLET and WAKSMAN (1966) were able to transfer tolerance to CBA skin in neonatally thymectomized A strain mice by transplanting thymic tissue or by injecting thymus cells from A mice which had been made tolerant to CBA cells. Grafts of normal thymus or injection of normal thymus cells restored the ability of these thymectomized animals to reject CBA skin homografts. Similar results have also been reported by ARGYRIS (1965). FOLLET et al. (1966), however, were able to induce tolerance to picrylchloride in adult thymectomized Hartley strain guinea pigs, and they concluded that the thymus need not be present for either induction or maintenance of tolerance to defined haptens in the adult animal.

To test the hypothesis that presence of the thymus is necessary for both recognition of "foreignness" (BURNET, 1962) and induction of tolerance (NOSSAL and MITCHELL, 1966; ISAKOVIC et al., 1965; TOULLET and WAKSMAN, 1966), attempts were made to induce tolerance to tetanus toxoid in normal and thymectomized mice (HESS and STONER, 1967 a, b).

Newborn mice of the BNL strain were given either a single injection, or a series of injections over a period of up to 5 weeks, of concentrated FTT, APTT, or toxin complexed at equivalence with isologous antitoxin. All animals responded to neonatal antigenic stimulation, regardless of the physical form of the antigen; there was no evidence of specific antigenic tolerance (Table 6).

Table 6. *Tetanus antitoxin responses in normal BNL-Swiss mice following neonatal injection of tetanus toxoid*

Physical form of antigen	Time and number of injections [a]	Total dose	Mean titers expressed as I.U. antitoxin/ml serum [b]	
			4 weeks after birth	3 weeks after challenge [c]
FTT [d] 5×conc.	single neonatal injection	0.05 ml	0.004	0.158
10×conc.	single neonatal injection	0.02 ml	0.004	0.338
10×conc.	4 injections within first week after birth	0.08 ml	0.008	0.500
10×conc.	11 injections within first 4 weeks	0.12 ml	3.250	9.375
APTT	single neonatal injection	0.02 ml	0.005	1.250
	4 injections within first week after birth	0.08 ml	0.175	2.000
	11 injections within first 4 weeks	0.12 ml	3.750	10.625
Active tetanus toxin in complex with isologous antitoxin at equivalence [e]	single neonatal injection	1,600 M.L.D.	0.0015	0.005
	4 injections within first week after birth	6,400 M.L.D.	0.002	0.675
	11 injections within first 4 weeks	17,600 M.L.D.	0.0156	7.375

[a] All injections given by intra-abdominal route

[c] 0.05 ml APTT by subcutaneous route at 4 weeks of age

[e] Dose given as M.L.D. of active toxin in complex

[b] 15 to 20 animals per group

[d] Fluid tetanus toxoid concentrated by evaporation

Table 7. *Tetanus antitoxin responses in neonatally thymectomized BNL-Swiss mice following neonatal antigen injection*

Experimental group (15—20 animals)	Antigen	Time and number of injections [a]	Total dose	Mean titers expressed as I.U. antitoxin/ml serum	
				4 weeks after birth	3 weeks after challenge [b]
Thymectomized	FTT [c] 5×conc.	Single neonatal injection	0.05 ml	0.003	0.100
Shamoperated	FTT 5×conc.	Single neonatal injection	0.05 ml	0.005	0.150
Thymectomized	Active tetanus toxin in complex with isologous antitoxin at equivalence [d]	Single neonatal injection	1,600 M.L.D.	0.0015	0.005
		4 injections within first week after birth	6,400 M.L.D.	0.002	0.625
Thymectomized controls (no neonatal injection)				0	0.0013
Normal controls (no neonatal injection)				0	0.003

[a] All injections given by intra-abdominal route

[c] Fluid tetanus toxoid concentrated by evaporation

[b] 0.05 ml APTT by subcutaneous route at 4 weeks of age

[d] Dose given as M.L.D. of active toxin in complex

Neonatal thymectomy, performed either before or after a single injection of concentrated FTT, or before single or multiple injections of complexed toxin in various doses, neither induced tolerance nor were the antitoxin titers produced higher than those of nonoperated controls (Table 7).

These observations indicate that tetanus toxoid is recognized as "foreign" even in the absence of the thymus. Furthermore, cells with the potential for producing tetanus antitoxin either were already present in sufficient numbers at the time of thymectomy, or, in case some of the responding cells were newly formed, apparently do not need the presence of the thymus in the course of their maturation. Before the possible role of the thymus in acquired immunological tolerance may be elucidated, the mechanisms involved in the tolerant state have to be analyzed more completely.

5. Additional Examples of Acquired Immunity in Thymectomized Animals

5.1. Hypersensitivity Reactions

The effect of neonatal thymectomy in mice on the development of immediate and delayed skin reactions was studied by RUSSE and CROWLE (1965). CF_1 mice were either thymectomized within 24 hours after birth or treated with daily intraperitoneal injections of rabbit antimouse thymic lymphocyte serum for a period of 24 to 84 days; at the age of 4 to 6 weeks, these animals were given two weekly sensitizing injections of ovalbumin or BSA in complete Freund's adjuvant. Thymectomized and serum-treated animals only developed severely impaired immediate and delayed hypersensitivity to these antigens as compared to nonoperated controls. This impairment, however, was temporary in both groups since upon reinjection of the sensitizing antigen or when sensitization was started at the age of 6 months, no difference was found between skin reactions of thymectomized, serumtreated, or nontreated mice.

Sprague-Dawley rats, when thymectomized at birth, exhibited severely depressed immediate and delayed hypersensitivity to BSA following sensitization at the age of 7 to 10 weeks; depression or absence of Arthus reactions were observed only in animals with impaired humoral antibody formation. Tuberculin sensitivity, tested at the same time intervals and measured on the basis of diameter and degree of skin lesions, was also considerably reduced in thymectomized rats as compared to nonoperated controls (ARNASON and JANKOVIC, 1962; JANKOVIC et al., 1962; ARNASON et al., 1962 b, c, 1964 b).

The same authors reported that thymectomy in Sprague-Dawley rats and Hartley strain guinea pigs at 2 to 3 weeks of age had no effect on the development of delayed hypersensitivity to BSA and ovalbumin (ARNASON and JANKOVIC, 1962; JANKOVIC et al., 1962). In a more recent report, BART et al. (1966) found no difference between neonatally thymectomized, sham-operated or nonoperated Hartley strain guinea pigs in development of contact sensitization to dinitrochlorobenzene.

Neonatally thymectomized Sprague-Dawley rats, inoculated with larvae of an intestinal nematode *(Nippostrongylus brasiliensis)* by subcutaneous route, were observed to form less antibody, measured by passive cutaneous anaphylaxis, than shamoperated controls. Despite low antibody titers practically no worm eggs were passed in the feces of thymectomized animals following re-inoculation, indicating that thymectomy did not interfere with the establishment of immunity not mediated by humoral antibody (R. J. M. WILSON et al., 1967).

Whereas the induction of "allergic encephalomyelitis" following injection of rat or guinea pig spinal cord in complete Freund's adjuvant was suppressed in the majority of neonatally thymectomized Sprague-Dawley or Lewis rats (ARNASON et al., 1962 a, b; DEFENDI et al., 1964), neonatal thymectomy did not appear to have any marked effects on the incidence of "adjuvant arthritis" which could be observed in about 40 to 50% of thymectomized and control Sprague-Dawley rats following footpad injection of complete Freund's adjuvant only (ARNASON et al., 1962 b, 1964 b); it should be noted that "adjuvant arthritis" may not necessarily be a specific immunologic process.

In addition, patients suffering from Swiss type agammaglobulinemia among other immunological defects, regularly exhibit inability to develop delayed hypersensitivity to various antigens and chemicals (see COTTIER et al., 1967); in one of these patients the inability to become sensitized to dinitrochlorobenzone could not be corrected by implants of fetal thymus or by injection of fetal liver cells (HITZIG et al., 1965).

It appears, therefore, that under certain conditions thymectomy in mammals may interfere with the ability to develop delayed hypersensitivity responses. This deficiency observed in neonatally thymectomized animals is more quantitative than qualitative: hypersensitivity reactions are, as a rule, not observed to be absent but diminished. The close relationship between depressed hypersensitivity reactions and the degree of peripheral lymphopenia, and, in some cases, the degree of impairment of humoral antibody formation may point to cellular *and* humoral mechanisms involved in delayed hypersensitive states.

5.2. Transplantation Immunity

The ability of mice to reject skin homografts was the first and most widely used test system in evaluating the effects of neonatal thymectomy on immune responsiveness. MILLER (1961) reported that 5 out of 7 neonatally thymectomized C3H mice "permanently" (from 45 to 101 days) accepted skin from Ak mice, and that 4 out of 6 thymectomized Ak mice, as well as all thymectomized (Ak×T6)F$_1$ hybrid mice accepted C3H skin for from 40 to 118 days. Deficient homograft rejection mechanisms were evident already at the age of 3 days in neonatally thymectomized mice while shamoperated littermates were able to reject skin grafts at that age (MILLER, 1964 b). This finding of severely impaired homograft rejection in neonatally thymectomized, conventionally raised mice has been confirmed in numerous strains using a variety of donor-host combinations. A synopsis of these results is presented in Table 8.

It may be worthwhile to emphasize the following:

1) Rejection time in thymectomized mice was usually, but not always (BASCH, 1966; BROOKE, 1965), prolonged; the "permanent" takes observed by MILLER (1962 b) are exceptional.

2) The occurence of post-thymectomy wasting appears to influence homograft rejection mechanisms much in the same way as humoral antibody formation. A number of "permanent takes" are based on the observation of animals dying from wasting disease with intact skin grafts. The ability of neonatally thymectomized, specific pathogen-free Swiss mice to reject 129/J strain skin was not impaired when tested at the age of 25 weeks. Even more important is the observation that only 5 out of 20 neonatally thymectomized germfree C57BL mice had rejection times exceeding 20 days for Balb/c skin (McINTIRE et al., 1962).

Adult thymectomy in mice was effective in impairing skin graft rejection across weak histocompatibility barriers, but had no influence on immune responses to stronger transplantation antigens. Thus, MARTINEZ et al. (1962 a) and GOOD et al. (1962) observed acceptance of Ce mouse skin grafts by adult thymectomized C3H mice; although both Ce and C3H mice belong to the H-2^k histocompatibility subgroup, control C3H mice were able to reject Ce mouse skin. Strong H-2 and sex-linked histocompatibility differences could not be overcome by adult thymectomy alone.

Adult thymectomy in combination with either sublethal or lethal irradiation and subsequent protection by bone marrow or fetal liver cells had a marked depressive effect on graft rejection mechanisms; protection of lethally irradiated thymectomized animals with adult, isologous spleen cells restored their ability to reject skin grafts within time intervals similar to those observed in normal animals (MILLER, 1962 a; MILLER et al., 1963; CROSS et al., 1964; GOEDBLOED and VOS, 1965). The effect of immunosuppressive therapy on homograft rejection in mice was not markedly potentiated when combined with adult thymectomy. Adult C3H mice were thymectomized, pretreated with different doses of cyclophosphamide, azathioprine or cortisone acetate, and grafted with AKI skin; adult thymectomy slightly prolonged skin graft survival only in animals which had received multiple injections of the immunosuppressive drugs over a period of several weeks (DUKOR and DIETRICH, 1967).

Impairment of skin homograft rejection following thymectomy has also been studied in species other than mice. Neonatally thymectomized Sprague-Dawley rats exhibited delayed onset and reduced speed of rejection of Sherwood strain rat skin over an observation period of 10 to 25 days (ARNASON et al., 1962 b, 1964 b). FISHER and FISHER (1965) reported on strain differences in skin graft rejection by thymectomized rats: while from 32 to 40% of Long-Evans strain rats, grafted at the age of one to 2 months with Sprague-Dawley skin, retained the grafts for more than 30 days, only approximately 6% of Sprague-Dawley rats took longer than 30 days to reject Long-Evans skin. Second-set skin grafts were tolerated exclusively by those animals in which rejection times for primary grafts exceeded 30 days. The ability of Lewis rats to reject BN-rat skin, on the other hand, was not affected by neonatal thymectomy (DEFENDI et al., 1964).

Homotransplantation immunity in rabbits, thymectomized before the age of 5 days, was not impaired (GOOD et al., 1962).

SHERMAN et al. (1962) reported that thymectomy in hamsters, even when performed as late as 2 weeks after birth, still effectively repressed the capacity to reject skin grafts from AJAX mice. On the other hand, it has been observed that the ability of Lakeview hamsters to reject skin from the isogenic CB strain was, at the most, moderately impaired, and that the operation had to be carried out within 6 to 24 hours after birth to be effective at all (ROOSA et al., 1965); in addition, these authors found a remarkable impairment of second-set graft rejection in hamsters thymectomized within 24 hours after birth.

Organ transplantation following thymectomy in combination with whole-body irradiation, splenectomy and immunosuppressive therapy was first attempted in 5 patients undergoing renal transplantation (STARZL et al., 1963). Despite severe signs of rejection from 15 to 27 days after the operation, 3 patients with transplants from unrelated donors had functioning kidneys for time periods ranging from 105 to 198 days. Evidence for beneficial effects of thymectomy in combination with immunosuppressive therapy in treatment of patients with renal transplants is inconclusive and difficult to assess (STARZL et al., 1965).

Kidney transplants in thymectomized dogs failed to be tolerated (FISHER et al., 1965); even when combined with chemotherapy, thymectomy in adult dogs did not prolong the survival of renal homografts beyond survival times observed following immunosuppressive therapy alone (CALNE, 1963).

Tumor transplantation across the strong H-2 histocompatibility barrier appears to be facilitated in neonatally thymectomized animals. MARTINEZ et al. (1962 b) and GOOD et al. (1962) observed that a mammary adeno-

Table 8. *Skin homograft rejection in neonatally thymectomized mice*

Thymectomized recipient	Wasting	Donor strain	Histocompatibility difference	Rejection time Nr. accepted/total Nr.	Authors
DBA/2	yes	(Balb/c×DBA/2)F₁	not H-2	27/27 longer than 28 d.	GOOD et al., 1962
				17/27 "permanently" [a]	
		C3H	H-2	9/12 longer than 35 d.	MARTINEZ et al., 1964
C3H	yes	(A×C3H)F₁	H-2	12/14 longer than 35 d.	MARTINEZ et al., 1964
		Ak	H-2	8/9 longer than 50 d.	MILLER, 1961
		Balb/c	H-2	5/7 longer than 50 d.	MILLER and DUKOR, 1964
		Rat	xenogeneic	3/6 longer than 25 d.	
Ak	yes	C3H	H-2	4/6 from 40 to 118 d.	MILLER, 1961
(Ak×T6)F₁	yes	C3H	H-2	18/25 longer than 50 d.	
		C57BL	H-2	9/15 longer than 50 d.	
		Balb/c	H-2	9/15 longer than 50 d.	MILLER and DUKOR, 1964
		DBA/2	H-2	4/14 longer than 50 d.	
		Rat	xenogeneic	7/16 longer than 25 d.	
C57BL	yes	Balb/c	H-2	"prolongation"	BASCH, 1966
		CBA	H-2	4/6 longer than 50 d. [a]	
		(DBA/2×C57BL)F₁	H-2	3/3 longer than 50 d. [a]	GOEDBLOED and VOS, 1965
		Rat	xenogeneic	3/3 longer than 50 d. [a]	

Table 8 (continued)

Thymectomized recipient	Wasting	Donor strain	Histocompatibility difference	Rejection time (Nr. accepted/total Nr.)	Authors
C57BL Females	yes	C57BL Males	Y-linked (EICHWALD-SILMSER)	6/6 longer than 35 d.	GOOD et al., 1962
C57BL/6J	(yes)	A/J	H-2	No difference between thymectomized and shamoperated	BROOKE, 1965
(RF×C57BL)F$_1$	yes	CBA	H-2	7/17 longer than 50 d. [a]	GOEDBLOED and VOS, 1965
		(CBA×C57BL)F$_1$	H-2	6/12 longer than 50 d. [a]	
		(DBA/2×C57BL)F$_1$	H-2	5/12 longer than 50 d. [a]	
		Rat	xenogeneic	3/12 longer than 50 d. [a]	
SL	yes	C57BL	H-2	11/18 longer than 60 d. [a]	TAKEYA and NOMOTO, 1967
LAF$_1$	yes	C3H	H-2	5/7 longer than 30 d.	SCHOOLEY et al., 1965
BNL-Swiss (specific pathogen-free)	no	129/J	?	No difference between thymectomized and shamoperated	HESS and STONER, 1967 b
C57BL (germfree)	no	Balb/c	H-2	5/20 longer than 20 d.	McINTIRE et al., 1964

[a] or died with intact graft

carcinoma, originating in A strain mice, was growing progressively in neo-natally thymectomized C3H mice whereas the tumor was regularly rejected by sham- or nonoperated controls.

However, neonatally thymectomized germfree CFW or C3H mice were demonstrated to have perfectly intact rejection mechanisms of homologous tumor transplants which were induced by methylcholanthrene in the other strain; only one out of 4 C3H mice accepted CFW transplants. Some tumor grafts remained intact when the neonatally thymectomized animals were irradiated before transplantation (BEALMEAR and WILSON, 1967 a).

Tumor graft acceptance could also be achieved by combined thymectomy and radiation treatment in adult conventional C57BL mice: sarcoma B-3, originating in male C57BL mice and regularly rejected by intact female mice of the same strain, grew progressively when the female recipients were thymectomized and subjected to a single dose of 550 r sublethal X-radia-tion. Sarcoma SBL-5, originating in H-2^b C57BL mice, was accepted by H-2^k C3H mice which were thymectomized and irradiated 7 days before transplantation; the tumor did not take in nontreated C3H controls (FELD-MAN and GLOBERSON, 1964).

Conflicting observations have been reported in rats: while PERRI et al. (1963) found progressive growth of Jensen sarcoma across the H-2 histo-compatibility barrier in thymectomized Sprague-Dawley rats, FISHER and FISHER (1965) found no difference in the rejection of Walker tumor tissue between neonatally thymectomized and nonoperated Long-Evans rats. Suc-cessful growth of a mammotropic tumor (MtT/F_4) was reported in neo-natally thymectomized, histoincompatible rats (LAZAR, 1966).

5.3. Graft-versus-host Reactions

Graft-versus-host (g.v.h.) assays were used in testing 1) the immuno-logical competence of lymphoid cells from thymectomized animals as measured by their ability to induce g.v.h. reactions in selected hosts, and 2) the immunological competence of thymectomized animals as measured by their ability to withstand the attack of lymphoid cells of a competent donor.

It has been shown that lymphoid cells of neonatally thymectomized animals exhibit a strikingly reduced capacity to induce g.v.h. reactions in adequate recipients as compared to lymphoid cells from normal animals (DALMASSO et al., 1962; MILLER and HOWARD, 1964; YUNIS et al., 1965). On the other hand, it appears that neonatal thymectomy might render mice more susceptible to the induction of g.v.h. runting (MARTINEZ et al., 1962 c; PARROT and EAST, 1964; McINTIRE et al., 1964).

DALMASSO et al. (1962) reported that spleen or lymph node cells of $(A \times C3H)F_1$ mice, thymectomized either at birth or at the age of up to

35 days, were unable to elicit g.v.h. reactions in newborn A strain mice recipients. Lymph node cells of thymectomized animals had to be injected in doses of up to 4 times the number of cells from normal controls in order to induce g.v.h. changes (MILLER, 1963). This apparent deficiency of lymphoid cells in thymectomized animals could be corrected by the injection of 10 to 100×10^6 adult spleen cells or of 100 to 400×10^6 neonatal or adult thymus cells; by the use of an allogeneic host-donor combination, it could be demonstrated that the lymphoid cells, active in eliciting g.v.h. reactions, of these reconstituted mice were of donor origin (YUNIS et al., 1965). Delayed effects of thymectomy in adult mice were observed also in g.v.h. assays: the ability of lymphoid cells from adult thymectomized CBA mice to induce spleen enlargement in young $(C57BL\times CBA)F_1$ hybrids was un-impaired for 25 weeks after the operation; at that age a sharp drop in g.v.h.-inducing capacities was noted which could only be attributed in part to the decreased cellularity of the lymphoid tissue (TAYLOR, 1965). Identical results were obtained by MILLER (1965 a) in the combination of adult thymectomized C3H and $(C3H\times C57BL)F_1$ mice. It appears doubtful that more can be gained from these experiments than evidence for a quantitative deficit in immunologically competent cells in thymectomized animals.

MARTINEZ et al. (1962 a) observed that thymectomy immediately after birth or at the age of 40 days increased the susceptibility of $(A\times C3H)F_1$ mice to the induction of g.v.h. runting by the injection of parental (A strain) cells, although C3H cells were ineffective. However, neither increase nor decrease in the intensity of g.v.h. reactions were described in Sprague-Dawley rats which were thymectomized at the age of 3 days and injected with spleen cells from Long-Evans rats (AISENBERG et al., 1962).

The observation of PARROT and EAST (1964) that postthymectomy wasting in C3H/Bi mice could be exacerbated by an intraperitoneal injection of 2×10^7 C57BL spleen cells was taken as confirmation of the hypothesis, first formulated by MILLER (1962 b) and PARROT and EAST (1962), that postthymectomy wasting may be etiologically related to g.v.h. runting. This hypothesis, however, has been cast into considerable doubt by the recent evidence of the role played by infectious processes in the induction of wasting disease (AZAR et al., 1964; WILSON et al., 1964 a, b; McINTIRE et al., 1964; BEALMEAR and WILSON, 1967 a).

6. Thymectomy and Bursectomy in Birds

The early reports of CHANG et al. (1955) and GLICK et al. (1956) that bursectomy in young chickens caused pronounced defects in antibody production in adult birds was based on a chance observation. For the production of antiserum against *Salmonella typhimurium* O-antigen some chickens were immunized which had been bursectomized in the course of another experiment; six out of these nine birds died immediately after antigen injection, and the three survivors did not produce agglutinating antibodies while nonoperated birds in the group produced normal antibody titers. In a controlled experiment, GLICK et al. showed that following bursectomy at 2 weeks of age and stimulation at 11 to 14 weeks later, only 8 out of a total of 75 birds produced agglutinins as compared to 63 responders out of 73 controls. Subsequently, MEYER et al. (1959) and MUELLER et al. (1960) reported that the development of the bursa could be arrested or inhibited by treatment of the fertilized egg with testosterone, and that birds with hormonally inhibited bursa development were unable to produce precipitins following stimulation with BSA at the age of 6 or 20 weeks. MUELLER et al. (1960) also found that surgical bursectomy as late as one or 2 weeks after hatching still repressed anti-BSA antibody formation, while bursectomy in chickens older than 5 weeks was without effect.

THORBECKE et al. (1957) had shown that the histology of the bursa of germfree and conventional chickens was not markedly different, and that bursa development and involution occurred at the same time in both groups. Based on these findings and on their own observation of defective antibody formation in bursaless birds, MUELLER et al. (1960) suggested that the bursa was a primary lymphoid organ in birds, necessary for the development of immune responsiveness, but not itself a site of immune reactions.

Absence or severe impairment of antibody formation in surgically or hormonally "bursectomized" birds following stimulation with antigens such as BSA, human gammaglobulin, *Leptospira icterohaemorrhagica*, *Brucella suis* or *abortus*, *Salmonella adelaide*, T2 coliphage, and influenza A virus, was also reported by WARNER et al. (1962), PAPERMASTER et al. (1962 b), KEMENES and PERTHES (1963), MUELLER et al. (1964), WARNER and SZENBERG (1964), and OKUYAMA (1965 a).

However, bursectomized chickens reportedly are able to produce gammaglobulin (PIERCE et al., 1966), and the formation of normal isoagglutinins is not affected by bursectomy (SOLOMON, 1966). An increased formation of IgM and an impaired production of IgG have been described by CAREY and WARNER (1964) and by COOPER et al. (1966 a). These findings led CLAFLIN et al. (1966) to reexamine the ability of hormone-treated chickens to produce antibody following stimulation with *Brucella abortus*. With the use of a sensitive method, these authors detected measurable and slightly depressed IgM-antibody responses and severely impaired IgG-antibody formation in these bursa-less birds. It should be noted that the hormone dose used by CLAFLIN et al. for suppression of bursa development was small enough to avoid atrophy of the thymic cortex.

Surgical bursectomy had no effect on homograft immunity, whereas surgical thymectomy at the time of hatching caused considerable delay in homograft rejection. Birds in which hormone-treatment during embryo-genesis had caused not only arrest of bursa development but also atrophy of the thymic cortex, died with intact grafts at from 7 to 24 days after skin transplantation (SZENBERG and WARNER, 1962 a; WARNER and SZENBERG, 1964). Similar results are reported by ASPINALL et al. (1963).

In graft-versus-host (g.v.h.) assays, no difference was observed by WARNER and SZENBERG (1963) in the reaction of newly hatched bursa-less chickens and normal controls following an injection of adult spleen cells; an impairment of bursa-less birds to counteract the attack of adult spleen cells was noted only when the injection was given at 12 days after hatching. However, PAPERMASTER et al. (1962 c) found bursa-less chickens to be far more susceptible to the induction of g.v.h. splenomegaly when the injection of adult spleen cells was administered at the age of 12 days. While spleen cells of 4-month-old bursa-less chickens were capable of producing g.v.h.-reactions in normal one-day-old recipients (WARNER and SZENBERG, 1963), COOPER et al. (1966 a) found that lymphoid cells from thymectomized birds were defective in producing splenomegaly upon injection into newly hatched chickens. In a different type of g.v.h.-assay, WARNER and SZENBERG (1964; SZENBERG and WARNER, 1962 a) tested the ability of peripheral blood or spleen cells to induce lesions on the chorioallantoic membrane (CAM) of 12-day-old chick embryos (*Simonsen* phenomenon), an immune reaction which supposedly is mediated by large and medium-sized lympho-cytes (SZENBERG and WARNER, 1962 b). CAM lesions could be produced by cells of both bursectomized and thymectomized birds.

Delayed hypersensitivity reactions to tuberculin and vaccinia virus were tested in normal, bursa-less and surgically thymectomized chickens. Whereas the normal and thymectomized animals developed typical skin reactions, bursa-less birds failed to react upon reexposure to the antigens (SZENBERG and WARNER, 1962 a; WARNER and SZENBERG, 1964). This finding is in contrast to observations made by OKUYAMA (1965 b) who found no defi-ciency in bursectomized chickens to develop delayed hypersensitivity to a heat-killed avian mycobacterium. COOPER et al. (1965, 1966 a, 1967) added whole-body irradiation to surgical thymectomy and/or bursectomy in newly hatched chickens. Thymectomized-irradiated birds had normal levels of immunoglobulins, but displayed deficient antibody responses to *Brucella abortus* and BSA, showed impairment of homograft rejection, delayed hypersensitivity and g.v.h.-reactions; a deficit of small lymphocytes was found in the circulating blood and in the white pulp of the spleen while germinal center formation and plasma cell production appeared to remain intact. In contrast, bursectomized-irradiated chickens were agammaglobu-linemic (lack of both 19 S- and 7 S-gammaglobulins) and were unable to produce humoral antibody following stimulation with *Brucella* or BSA, while homograft rejection mechanisms and the ability to produce g.v.h.-

reactions were not impaired; in these animals both germinal center and plasma cell formation were rare or absent.

Based on these observations, COOPER et al. (1966 a)proposed the existence in birds of two cell populations with distinct immunologic competence, one dependent on the presence of the bursa, the other thymus-dependent, a concept which had been put forward already by WARNER et al. (1962). But whereas WARNER et al. found the development of delayed hypersensitivity reactions to be dependent on the bursa and even proposed a third population of cells of unknown origin as precursors for the CAM lesion-producing cells (WARNER and SZENBERG, 1964), according to COOPER et al. (1966 a, 1967) cells derived from the avian thymus would be instrumental in expressions of "cellular immunity" (including delayed hypersensitivity, homograft rejection and g.v.h.-reactivity); bursa-derived cells would be mainly concerned with germinal center formation and immunoglobulin production. In fact, restoration of immunoglobulin and germinal center formation was observed in bursectomized-irradiated chickens which were reinjected with their own dispersed bursa cells; however, these reconstituted birds were still unable to produce specific antibodies to BSA and *Brucella* antigens (COOPER et al., 1966 b).

Several points may be raised to question the overall validity of this concept: 1) It should be emphasized that testosterone treatment of the chick embryo not only arrests bursa development but also causes atrophy of the thymic cortex in at least 30% of the animals (WARNER and SZENBERG, 1964), and may also be responsible for underdevelopment of other lymphoid tissues not directly related to the bursa; an interdependence of thymus and bursa cannot be excluded by experiments based on extirpation combined with whole-body irradiation since radiation damage to the remaining organ certainly occurs, as witnessed by the significantly shortened lifespan of bursectomized-irradiated birds. 2) Hormonal arrest of bursa development in doses which do not cause morphologically visible damage to the thymus cortex does not preclude antibody formation by the adult bird (CLAFLIN et al., 1966). 3) It is still unsettled whether delayed hypersensitivity reactions depend (COOPER et al., 1966 a) or do not depend (WARNER and SZENBERG, 1964) in part, or entirely, on the presence of the thymus. 4) Recent observations by ISAKOVIC and JANKOVIC (1967) indicate that following hyperimmunization even in the absence of the bursa germinal center and plasma cell formation may occur, and that both 7S- and 19S-antibody are produced.

This concept of a dissociation in the development of immune responsiveness, inspite of these incertainties, has gained considerable attention since the hypothesis of a similar dichotomy in the development of immunity in mammals has been proposed by GOOD's group (ARCHER et al., 1964 a, b; SUTHERLAND et al., 1964; GOOD et al., 1966 b; COOPER et al., 1967). The much searched-for bursa-equivalent in mammals has not been clearly defined (COOPER et al., 1966 c); nevertheless, GOOD's hypothesis has been used in classifying immune deficiency syndromes in man (GOOD et al., 1967; COTTIER et al., 1967), and its chief merit appears to lie in stimulating clinical studies of these poorly understood disorders.

7. Post-thymectomy Wasting

In the first studies on the effect of neonatal thymectomy in mice it has been observed that operated animals showed normal body growth only during a period lasting from several weeks to a few months. After that period of good health, thymectomized animals became sick with what was termed "post-thymectomy wasting syndrome"; in contrast to sham- or non-operated control animals, wasting mice stopped to gain weight and developed a characteristically hunched posture, their fur became ruffled, then they lost weight, developed diarrhea, and most died within 60 to 90 days of the operation (PARROT, 1962; MILLER, 1963).

Wasting has been reported to occur in a great number of conventionally raised mouse strains at various time intervals after neonatal thymectomy (Table 9). BALNER and DERSJANT (1966) observed a sex-difference in the incidence of wasting in neonatally thymectomized C57BL or (CBA×C57BL)F$_1$ mice: whereas 21 out of 44 males died within 6 months after the operation, only 9 out of 35 females succumbed to fatal wasting during the same period of time. No sex-differences have been noted by other investigators working with the same strains of mice. Thymectomy performed in mice older than 6 days (HILGARD et al., 1964 a), even when combined with whole-body irradiation (MILLER et al., 1964) was not followed by wasting. Similar to the observation by BARNES et al. (1964), BAZIN and DUPLAN (1967) reported on the occurrence of wasting in adult thymectomized mice, exposed to a lethal dose of X-radiation and protected by the injection of fetal liver cells; no wasting was observed when the irradiated animals were protected with adult lymphoid cells.

In Sprague-Dawley, Lewis or CFN rats, post-thymectomy wasting usually affected only from 10 to 30% of all animals (ARNASON et al., 1962 b, 1964 b; AZAR et al., 1964; PERRI et al., 1963; PINNAS and FITCH, 1966), and was sometimes confined to single cages (ISAKOVIC et al., 1965). However, in the hands of FISHER and FISHER (1965), neonatally thymectomized, conventionally raised Sprague-Dawley and Long-Evans rats were not affected by wasting.

Whereas post-thymectomy wasting was observed in rabbits only following neonatal thymectomy combined with appendectomy (SUTHERLAND et al., 1965) or after adult thymectomy combined with whole-body irradiation

Table 9. *Occurrence of post-thymectomy wasting in neonatally thymectomized conventional mice*

Strain	Onset of disease	Course	Authors
AKR	about 4 weeks	100% dead between 21—83 days	Parrot and East, 1964
TO	about 4 weeks	100% dead between 31—64 days if thymectomized within 12 hours after birth; 10% dead at 52 days if thymectomized between 12 to 24 hours after birth	Parrot and East, 1964
C57BL	4 weeks	100% dead between 30—39 days	Parrot and East, 1964
	4 weeks	100% dead at 50 days	Miller, 1963
	3—5 weeks	87% dead at 76 days	Basch, 1966
	7 weeks	60% sick or dead at 90 days; males more affected than females	Balner and Dersjant, 1966
	?	52% dead between 39—125 days	Law et al., 1964
	3 weeks	?	Dalmasso et al., 1962
C3H	about 4 weeks	100% dead between 29—64 days	Parrot and East, 1964
	about 3 weeks	90% dead between 38—74 days	Dalmasso et al., 1962
	?	68—85% dead between 30—148 days	Law et al., 1964
	7 weeks	75% dead at 120 days	Miller, 1963

Table 9 (continued)

Strain	Onset of disease	Course	Authors
(C57BL×C3H)F_1	about 4 weeks	100% dead between 27—113 days	Parrot and East, 1964
DBA/2	about 3 weeks	90% dead between 45—89 days	Dalmasso et al., 1962
	?	83% dead between 44—84 days	Law et al., 1964
(Ak×T6)F_1	6 weeks	75% dead at 120 days	Miller, 1963
CBA	?	80% dead within 126 days	Osoba, 1965 a
	7 weeks	50% sick at 90 days; no spontaneous deaths	De Vries et al., 1964
(CBA×T6)F_1	6 weeks	70% dead at 140 days	Osoba and Miller, 1964
(CBA×C57BL)F_1	7 weeks	50% sick or dead at 90 days; males more affected than females	Balner and Dersjant, 1966
A-Swiss	?	50% dead at 120 days	Rogister, 1964
Balb/c	?	23% dead between 80—95 days	Law et al., 1964
LAF_1	?	16% sick at 100 days	Schooley et al., 1965

(KELLUM and ECKERT, 1965), wasting commonly occurred in neonatally thymectomized hamsters. In the hamster strain used by SHERMAN et al. (1963) only male animals were affected by wasting, while no sex-difference in the incidence of wasting was reported by ROOSA et al. (1965). In guinea pigs, wasting was even described to occur 10 days after thymectomy in adult life (COMSA, 1957).

The most striking histopathological finding in thymectomized animals, whether suffering from wasting or apparently healthy, was a more or less severe scarcity of small lymphocytes in the peripheral blood and in lymphoid tissue (WAKSMAN et al., 1962; MILLER and DUKOR, 1964). This lymphopenia was found to be more pronounced in mice dying from wasting than in animals which were sacrificed as controls (DE VRIES et al., 1964). A detailed description of histopathological changes associated with post-thymectomy wasting in mice was presented by PARROT and EAST (1962), MILLER and DUKOR (1964) and DE VRIES et al. (1964). Lymph nodes were variable described as atrophic without germinal centers and plasma cells (MILLER and DUKOR, 1964) or as moderately to greatly enlarged with sometimes hyperplastic follicles (DE VRIES et al., 1964). Hyperplasia of reticulo-endothelial elements, especially in the sinusoids of the medulla was always noted. Similarly, hypoplasia of lymphoid elements and hyperplasia of reticulo-endothelial structures were observed in the spleen where the mass of the red pulp was found to be increased. Plasma cells could either not be found (PARROT and EAST, 1962; MILLER and DUKOR, 1964) or were present in great numbers (DE VRIES et al., 1964). Peyer's patches were small or absent, and small and large intestines exhibited signs of chronic inflammation. The bone marrow, including bone marrow lymphoid cells, remained unaffected by either thymectomy or wasting, except that in some cases an increased number of myeloblastic cells and/or small necrotic foci were described (DE VRIES et al., 1964). In the liver, hyperplasia of the reticulo-endothelial system (Kupffer cells) was noted repeatedly, and a large percentage of wasting mice had small necrotic lesions in the liver parenchyma (PARROT and EAST, 1962; MILLER and DUKOR, 1964). Phagocytic activity has been reported to be increased in neonatally thymectomized mice (SCHOOLEY et al., 1965) and rats (CORSI and GLUSTI, 1967); an impaired radiogold clearance was observed in adult thymectomized and irradiated Swiss mice (FRIDRICH and SCHÄFER, 1966).

In mice, no obvious evidence of specific infection could be found, but in neonatally thymectomized rats AZAR et al. (1964) noted mediastinal abscesses and bronchopneumonia in many animals; the incidence of wasting was reduced by 50% in neonatally thymectomized rats which were continously treated with tetracycline. LAW (1966 a) found no evidence for the presence in wasting mice of murine pneumonia virus, reovirus type 3, Theiler mouse encephalomyelitis virus (GDV II), Sendai virus, mouse pneumonitis K virus, or mouse hepatitis virus. EAST et al. (1963) were successful in isolating the hepatotrophic MHV-I virus from mice affected with wasting, and an occasional activation of latent infections with *Eperythrozoon coccoides* was reported in neonatally thymectomized mice (METCALF, 1966). Despite the scarcity of direct evidence, it appears very probable that the direct cause of wasting and death in neonatally thymectomized animals may result from systemic infection.

The view that post-thymectomy wasting has an infectious etiology is strongly supported not only by the fact that wasting was sometimes confined to single cages (ISAKOVIC et al., 1965), and that the incidence of wasting could be reduced by treatment with antibiotics (AZAR et al., 1964), but most of all by the observation that neither specific pathogen-free (HESS et al., 1963) nor germfree mice (WILSON et al., 1964 a, b; McINTIRE et al., 1964) exhibit signs of post-thymectomy wasting. Wasting could be easily induced in neonatally thymectomized germfree animals simply by transferring them from the germfree to a "conventional" environment. This constitutes conclusive evidence for the concept that wasting is caused by an infectious process which may eventually override the lowered resistance of thymectomized animals while not causing any apparent ill effects in non-operated animals. An increased susceptibility to infection and various toxins following thymectomy has been described in the old literature (KLOSE and VOGT, 1910; HELLMAN and WHITE, 1930); in more recent reports, decreased resistance of neonatally thymectomized mice and rats to coxsackie B, herpes simplex and 3 different adenoviruses (LEYTEN et al., 1965), decreased resistance to *Mycobacterium leprae* (REES, 1966), and increased susceptibility to endotoxin injection *(Escherichia coli, Salmonella typhi)* or to infection with *Candida albicans* or *tropicalis* (SALVIN et al., 1965) have been described. Multiple endotoxin injections (SALVIN et al., 1965), early infection with coxsackie B or herpes virus (LEYTEN et al., 1965) or intraperitoneal injection of complete Freund's adjuvant in mice (MORTON and SIEGEL, 1966) were sufficient to induce wasting in nonwasting neonatally thymectomized animals. Neonatally thymectomized rats, however, showed no increased susceptibility to endotoxin injection as compared to shamoperated controls (PORTER et al., 1966). A clinical syndrome, closely resembling post-thymectomy wasting in rodents, could be induced in adult thymectomized baboons by inoculation of adenovirus type 12 by various routes; no adenovirus could be isolated at the time of death (KALTER et al., 1967).

The fact that only animals thymectomized within the first 2 days after birth appear to be susceptible to wasting while animals kept in the same environment but operated upon at the age of 4 or more days are not affected at all may be explained by a decrease within that period of time of the permeability of the intestinal wall to the normal bacterial flora and to other infectious organisms. Another explanation could be based on the

hypothesis that at the age of a few days migration of a sufficient number
of cells to the periphery has already occurred, so that even in the absence
of the thymus the endogenous infectious process may be adequately checked.

An alternative hypothesis for the etiology of post-thymectomy wasting
has recently been advanced by DE VRIES et al. (1964). These authors observed that in neonatally thymectomized, conventional CBA/Rij, C57BL/Rij
or (CBA×C57BL)F₁ mice a retarded development of the lymphoid tissues
was followed by secondary atrophy. This atrophy of the lymphoid tissue
was found to be associated with histological changes in lymphoid and other
organs which, according to their view, could not be explained on the basis
of an infectious process. In the opinion of DE VRIES et al. these histopathological lesions were exhibiting some characteristics in common with lesions
encountered in g.v.h.-runting and, in addition, with lesions which may be
observed in cases of human lupus erythematosus. Based on this interpretation of the histopathological picture presented by wasting mice, it was
postulated that the post-thymectomy wasting syndrome may be caused
primarily by a lack of "self"-recognition of immunologically competent
cells. The lymphoid atrophy would be caused by an autoimmune process
which may proceed unchecked in the absence of the thymus (BURNET, 1962).
An attempt was made to resolve the difficult problem of reconciling this
proposed immune hyperactivity with the generally observed diminished
ability of thymectomized animals to respond to antigenic stimulation by
postulating preoccupation of lymphoid cells with anti-"self" reactivity.

Although in a series of reports the thymus has been linked to autoimmune processes, it has never been clearly resolved whether a pathological
function of the thymus plays an etiological role in autoimmune disease or
whether it may simply be one of several target organs, the observed thymus
changes being of secondary nature (see HOWIE and HELYER, 1966; HOLMES
and BURNET, 1966; STRAUSS and VAN DER GELD, 1966).

The fact remains that thymectomized pathogen-free or animals which
are largely protected from infectious agents neither develop signs of autoimmune processes nor wasting disease.

8. Morphological and Functional Lymphoid Reconstitution of Thymectomized Animals

Various attempts have been made to achieve reversal of morphological
and immunological defects in thymectomized animals. Early experiments by
MILLER (1961) proved subcutaneous grafts of thymic tissue to be successful
in preventing wasting disease and in restoring homograft immunity in neonatally thymectomized mice. Besides thymic grafts, injection of thymus,

spleen or lymph node lymphocytes, thymic tissue in cell-tight Millipore envelopes, and the administration of thymic extracts have been tested with varying success.

8.1. Thymus Implants

As early as 1950, LAW and J. H. MILLER (1950) demonstrated that the potentiality for lymphoma development could be restored by implanting syngeneic thymus grafts in DBA mice in which adult thymectomy had reduced the incidence of methylcholanthrene-induced leukemia. In similar fashion, it could be shown by KAPLAN that the incidence of radiation-induced lymphoid tumors in C57BL mice was reduced in thymectomized animals (KAPLAN, 1950) while lymphomas readily developed in thymectomized, irradiated mice carrying a thymus implant (KAPLAN and BROWN, 1954). GROSS (1959) and MILLER (1960) found that thymectomy performed at the age of 4 weeks prevented the development of leukemia in C3H mice which had been injected at birth with a cell-free leukemic filtrate; however, from 50 to 100% of these thymectomized animals developed leukemia when thymus lobes from normal, noninjected C3H mice were implanted as late as 6 months after thymectomy (MILLER, 1960).

Neonatally thymectomized $(Ak \times T6)F_1$ or $(C57BL \times T6)F_1$ mice which were grafted subcutaneously with parental (Ak and C57BL, respectively) or allogeneic (C3H, Ak or C57BL) thymic tissue from neonatal donors developed normally, had a normal life span, normal peripheral lymphocyte counts, and normally developed lymphoid tissue (MILLER, 1961, 1962 b). Thymectomized $(Ak \times T6)F_1$ mice, carrying Ak thymus grafts, rejected skin from allogeneic donors (C3H, C57BL, Balb/c, DBA/2) within 30 days, and they showed evidence of immunity to second-set grafts. When allogeneic thymus was implanted, skin graft rejection of thymus-donor skin was prolonged beyond 30 days in most cases, although third-party skin was rejected normally (MILLER, 1964 b). Restoration of homograft immunity by thymus grafts in either neonatally thymectomized or adult thymectomized, irradiated animals was reported also by GLOBERSON and FELDMAN (1964), FELDMAN and GLOBERSON (1964), RICHER et al. (1965), LEUCHARS et al. (1965), and MILLER (1966). Skin homograft immunity and the ability to produce anti-SRC antibodies could be restored in neonatally thymectomized $(C57BL \times C3H)F_1$ mice by either rat or hamster thymus grafts; wasting was "almost completely" prevented by these xenogeneic grafts, and the lymphoid tissues of the restored animals were not quite as depleted as in nontreated controls (LAW, 1966 b).

The finding that post-thymectomy wasting of neonatally thymectomized animals could be prevented by thymus grafts was confirmed by PARROT and EAST (1964); in the hands of these authors, thymic tissue placed under the kidney capsule was much more effective in preventing wasting disease than grafts implanted subcutaneously, and early grafting of young adult thymus was superior to implanting thymus tissue from older donors. It should be noted that wasting, once started, could not be reversed by single thymic implants (HILGARD et al., 1964 b; YUNIS et al., 1965); according to a recent report, however, reversal of wasting could be achieved when up to 5 thymic grafts were applied either subcutaneously or intra-abdominally (STUTMAN et al., 1967).

The mechanisms by which thymic grafts restore immune functions in thymectomized hosts are unknown. It may be pertinent to point out that a thymic graft, be it implanted subcutaneously, intraabdominally or under the kidney capsule, does not constitute a true replacement of an anatomically intact thymus with its lymph and blood vessels; nevertheless, grafted thymic tissue has been proposed to function very much like an intact thymus, and the following possibilities have been listed (MILLER, 1966): 1) The graft may provide cells which attain immunologic competence after migration to host lymphoid tissue. Very few thymus-derived cells, identified by a marker chromosome, were found in regional lymph nodes of thymectomized hosts (MILLER, 1966); however, LEUCHARS et al. (1964, 1966) observed a considerable increase in the number of thymus-derived cells in spleen and lymph nodes after antigenic stimulation of adult, thymectomized and irradiated mice carrying thymus implants. 2) The grafted thymus may provide primitive host cells with an environment in which they could acquire immunologic competence. In fact, there is abundant evidence that within 21 days after grafting nearly all dividing cells in the thymus implant are of host origin (MILLER, 1962 b; DALMASSO et al., 1963; METCALF, 1964; METCALF and WAKONIG-VAARTAJA, 1964; METCALF et al., 1965; DUKOR et al., 1965); however, thymic grafts have a restorative effect on immune capacity even when they are excised 10 days after implantation, i.e. at a time when a detectable host cell immigration was not yet observed (MILLER et al., 1966). 3) Grafted thymic tissue may also provide the host with (a) humoral and/or contact factor(s), inducing development of host lymphoid cells towards immunologic competence (MILLER, 1965 b, 1966). This last possibility remains hypothetical until such a factor has been isolated and found to be effective.

Based on these experimental findings, several attempts have been made in clinical studies at transferring thymus, liver homogenate or even tonsillar and gut-associated lymphoid tissue to patients suffering from immunologic deficiency diseases (ROSEN et al., 1962, 1966; GITLIN et al., 1964; ALLIBONE et al., 1965). These attempts were all unsuccessful. In the case of HITZIG et al. (1965), discussed in some detail by COTTIER et al. (1967), a baby girl suffering from Swiss type agammaglobulinemia was given a total of 3 infusions of fetal liver cells and was twice implanted with fetal thymus tissue. Despite questionable rises in the number of peripheral lymphocytes after each thymus implantation, the child died from an extensive, necrotizing pneumonia, and at autopsy no trace of lymphoid tissue was found in the spleen, in several lymph nodes and in the gut wall. In addition, no germinal centers were detectable, and the absence of plasma cells in the intestinal wall, in most lymph nodes, and in the spleen was noted. The first implanted thymus had disappeared under the formation of a lipogranuloma, with no signs of lymphocytic infiltration, and it was excised before the second implant was administered. The second thymus graft had survived in the child's abdominal wall for more than 10 months without any signs of inflammatory infiltrates. The Hassal's corpuscles were well developed and the lymphoid cell content considerably higher than in the child's own thymus. The bone marrow contained massive infiltrates of medium or large plasmocytoid cells. In view of the unexpected finding of pronounced plasmocytosis in the bone marrow in the absence of lymphoid parenchyma and plasma cells in other organs, the problem arises concerning the origin of the plasmocytoid cells in the bone marrow. This question could not be solved beyond doubt in this case, but several possibilities have been considered (COTTIER et al., 1967): the cells could either stem from the mother since XX/XY chimerism has been found in a condition related to Swiss type agammaglobulinemia (KADO-WAKI et al., 1965), or they could have been transferred with the grafted thymuses and/or liver suspensions although both were of fetal origin. The latter possibility seems more probable since no S-chromatin (*"Barr bodies"*) could be found in the bone marrow preplasmocytes. Synthesis of donor-type gammaglobulin following fetal thymus transplantation has recently been reported by HARBOE et al. (1966). Even if the cells stem from the implants it is still unresolved whether the cellular reaction observed in this case was the expression of a graft-versus-host reaction or a graft-versus-graft reaction in an immunologically unresponsive host. The exclusive localization of plasma cells in the bone marrow tends to favor the second possibility, since the bone marrow appears to be the most likely site where fetal hemopoietic tissue may home.

8.2. Injection of Lymphoid Cells

An intravenous injection of 5×10^6 dissociated thymus cells from a one-day-old donor mouse administered to a syngeneic recipient immediately after neonatal thymectomy failed to prevent impairment of homograft immunity or the development of wasting disease (MILLER, 1962 b, 1964 b). In the hands of ISAKOVIC et al. (1965), up to 10 to 20×10^8 thymus cells given to neonatally thymectomized rats during 4 or 8 weeks before immunization with BSA had no restorative effect on depressed antibody formation; lymph node cells were effective in conferring some immunologic recovery and in normalizing the level of circulating and lymph node lymphocytes.

TRAININ et al. (1965), however, achieved a significant reduction in the incidence of wasting disease when neonatally thymectomized C3H/Lw mice were given 1 to 3×10^7 thymus cells from newborn or adult donors one day after the operation; although peripheral lymphocyte counts remained below normal control values, some of the treated animals were able to respond to stimulation with SRC. The effectiveness of cell suspensions appears to depend largely on the number of cells administered. Neonatally thymectomized C3H and A mice when given total doses of 200 to 400×10^6 syngeneic (HILGARD et al., 1964 b) or allogeneic (YUNIS et al., 1964) thymus or spleen cells over a period of 2 to 3 weeks did not develop wasting disease, or, if the treatment was started after the onset of wasting, resumed normal body growth. Both syngeneic and allogeneic thymus and spleen cells were able to confer some degree of immunologic competence as judged by the ability of spleen cells from treated, thymectomized animals to elicit graft-versus-host reactions.

The effectiveness of cell suspensions in preventing or, with higher doses, even in reverting the post-thymectomy wasting syndrome may be explained as due to a direct supply of immunologically competent cells (TRAININ et al., 1965; HILGARD et al., 1964 b). The finding that lymph node or spleen cells were superior to thymus cells appears to support this hypothesis. The fact that bone marrow cells were effective to some degree in restoring immune functions in thymectomized mice (TRAININ et al., 1965) is hard to reconcile with the notion that bone marrow cells have to acquire immunologic competence by first passing through the thymus (LOUTIT, 1962; FORD et al., 1966).

It is also difficult to see how the concept of an autoimmune etiology of wasting (DE VRIES et al., 1964) should correlate with the results of these reconstitution experiments. Although lymphoid tissues, in general, were not found to be repopulated, and although a considerable number of deaths was noted among apparently reconstituted animals within an observation period of several months (TRAININ et al., 1965), wasting could be reversed by the supply of enough lymphoid cells in the absence of the thymus. A reversal of an autoimmune process by the administration of large numbers of immunologically competent cells appears to be highly improbable. In fact, it is more logical to assume that the administration of lymphoid cells at the right moment may just help the lymphopenic animals to overcome an otherwise fatal infection. It is not clear whether this support could also be explained by a trephocytic function of lymphoid cells (LOUTIT, 1962).

Finally, it should be pointed out that survival of equal numbers of transfused cells has to be assured before the relative capacity of these elements to restore immune deficiencies may be compared. To the best of our knowledge, no such studies have been made with regard to thymic vs. lymph node lymphoid cells.

8.3. Diffusion Chamber Implants Containing Lymphoid Cells

Results obtained in reconstitution of thymectomized animals with thymus tissue enclosed in cell-tight Millipore envelopes for many provided strong evidence in favor of a humoral function of the thymus.

Levey et al. (1963 a) reported that neonatally thymectomized Swiss-Webster mice were resistant to intracerebral inoculation of lymphocytic choriomeningitis (LCM) virus (CA 1371 strain) while all nonoperated controls died within 8 days of inoculation. The protective effect of thymectomy on subsequent LCM virus inoculation could be reduced by either subcutaneous grafting of a newborn thymus (6 out of 11 mice died) or by implanting a 0.45 μ pore size Millipore chamber containing a newborn thymus into the abdominal cavity (16 out of 31 mice died). Carriers of empty Millipore chambers behaved like thymectomized animals. The authors concluded that most probably the epithelial-reticular cells of the thymic implants produced a substance which stimulated lymphocyte production. This concept was further tested, and it was observed that neonatally thymectomized C3H/Lw and C3Hf/Bi mice when implanted with Millipore envelopes containing isologous newborn thymus developed no lymphopenia, no involution of lymphoid tissue and no wasting disease; thymectomized controls which had not been implanted with diffusion chambers died within 7 to 8 weeks with signs of severe wasting (Levey et al., 1963 b).

While Levey et al. (1963 a) reported on the occurrence of wasting even in reconstituted mice, Osoba and Miller (1963, 1964) absserved normal weight gain and practically no wasting within an observation period of 21 weeks in their neonatally thymectomized CBA or (CBA×T6)F$_1$ mice which were implanted with a 0.3 μ pore size Millipore envelope containing thymus tissue. Osoba and Miller described slight improvement of 1) peripheral lymphocyte counts in mice treated with either fetal or newborn thymus in diffusion chambers, 2) antibody formation against SRC, and 3) homograft rejection of Ak skin in thymectomized F$_1$ mice. Following implantation of thymus tissue in diffusion chambers, most of the lymph nodes (16 out of 23 examined) still had a deficient number of small lymphocytes in the cortical area; only occasional lymph nodes were rich in small lymphocytes and contained germinal centers and plasma cells. This finding is in marked contrast to the observation of Levey et al. (1963 b) who reported that thymectomized mice carrying Millipore implants had spleen, lymph nodes and, in particular, Peyer's patches "rich in lymphocytes"; there is, however, good correlation between this observation of lymphoid hyperplasia in the intestinal lymphoid tissue and the occurrence of wasting (de Vries et al., 1964).

The tissue in the diffusion chamber reportedly loses its lymphoid appearance within 10 days after implantation and is composed entirely of epithelial-reticular cells (OSOBA, 1965 a); there was no good correlation between the rise in body weight, extent of lymphoid repopulation and reconstitution of immune responsiveness (OSOBA and MILLER, 1964). These authors therefore suggested that "a humoral factor produced by the thymus epithelial-reticular complex may be responsible for endowing lymphoid cells with immunological competence".

These original observations on possible reconstitution of thymectomized animals with thymic tissue implanted in diffusion chambers have been extended by OSOBA (1965 a, b). Neonatally thymectomized CBA mice were implanted with 0.1 μ pore size Millipore envelopes containing adult axillary lymph nodes, adult or newborn spleen, or either syngeneic or allogeneic (C57BL) thymus. About 50% of mice implanted with either thymus tissue responded to stimulation with SRC, while animals carrying lymph node or spleen implants had severely impaired responses, comparable to those of thymectomized controls. Skin grafts from Ak mice were tolerated for more than 20 days by all thymectomized CBA mice, and also by animals carrying spleen or lymph node implants; in contrast, only 7 out of 21 mice with CBA thymus, and 2 out of 19 with C57BL thymus, had rejection times for Ak skin in excess of 40 days. While most of the thymectomized controls died from wasting within 18 weeks, fatal wasting was observed in only 50% of thymectomized mice with thymus, lymph node or spleen implants. Peripheral lymphocyte counts remained low, and no restoration of lymph node lymphocytes was observed. In another approach (1965 b), neonatally thymectomized, female CBA mice were mated with normal T6 males; after one to 2 litters, these females were found to have recovered some degree of immune reactivity. This finding was explained as being due to the action of a humoral thymic factor, produced by the fetal mice during pregnancy.

The question of cells escaping from the diffusion chamber, to our knowledge, has not been studied by the implantation of lymphoid tissue with a chromosome marker. However, evidence that chambers, at least with membrane pore sizes of from 0.1 to 0.01 μ, are cell-tight with regard to enclosed ascites tumor cells has been obtained; chambers with these pore sizes containing thymic tissue were still effective in restoring skin homograft rejection in adult, irradiated mice (BARCLAY et al., 1964).

Partial restoration of immune responsiveness by thymus-containing diffusion chambers has also been reported in rats (AISENBERG and WILKES, 1965; BIGGART, 1966 b), hamsters (WONG et al., 1966), and rabbits (TRENCH et al., 1966). It appears noteworthy to stress that in no instance a complete recovery of immunological competence had been achieved, and that neither lymphoid tissue nor peripheral lymphocytes were found to be normalized (BIGGART, 1966 a).

Of importance is also the observation of WONG et al. (1966) that restorative effects on anti-human gammaglobulin production in thymectomized hamsters could not only be achieved by implantation of diffusion chambers containing thymic tissue but, to a lesser extent, also with diffusion chambers containing bone marrow or kidney cells. The possibility of an "adjuvant effect" of Millipore diffusion chambers was disclaimed based on the finding that empty chambers or chambers containing necrotic tissue were ineffective. It may be noted, however, that in the report of WONG et al. humoral antibody formation of control animals with implanted thymus or other tissue was enhanced over responses elicited in non-implanted controls. It is conceivable that an equal "nonspecific" effect may be operative in thymectomized animals, enhancing depressed antibody responses which would otherwise remain below measurable titers.

8.4. Summary

Evidence of all these reconstitution experiments, though inconclusive, appears to support the notion that thymus epithelial cells may produce a humoral and/or contact factor with lymphopoiesis-stimulating properties (METCALF, 1956; OSOBA, 1966; CLARK, 1966). Considerable attention has been paid lately to the question of whether the PAS positive inclusions found in thymic epithelial cells may be an expression of the elaboration of such (a) substance(s) (ISHIDATE and METCALF, 1963; METCALF, 1964; CLARK, 1966). The possibility cannot be excluded that at least some of the PAS-positive cells in the thymus merely reflect degenerative processes since similar cells with similar tinctorial and histochemical properties may be found in other organs following tissue breakdown (COTTIER, 1961; DE VRIES, 1967).

In addition to the lymphopoiesis-stimulating property, a "competence-inducing" action has also been ascribed to the thymus (LEVEY et al., 1963 a; FELDMAN and GLOBERSON, 1964; MILLER, 1964 b, 1966). This "competence-inducing" factor has been described to induce differentiation of undifferentiated, incompetent lymphoid cells in the course of which they would acquire immunological competence. The evidence for the existence of such a substance also is inconclusive, and the question has not been settled whether close contact between lymphoid cells and thymus epithelial cells is required for its action, or whether it may also be effective at a distance.

A recent report on the isolation of a thymus-derived glycoprotein ("thymosin") with lymphopoietic properties (GOLDSTEIN et al., 1966) is just one of a series of attempts to isolate active substances from thymic tissue. Isolation attempts started when METCALF (1956) published his finding of a lymphocytosis-stimulating factor (LSF) in the thymus of leukemic mice (GREGOIRE and DUCHATEAU, 1956; CAMBLIN and BRIDGES, 1964; DE SOMER et al., 1963; COMSA, 1965; KLEIN et al., 1965, 1966; TRAININ et al., 1966; HAND et al., 1967).

None of these substances, presumably produced by the thymus, has been isolated in a satisfactory manner, and repetition of the isolation procedure almost always failed. Until reliable methods for the separation of a well-defined substance with reproduceable biological activity have been devised, the existence of humoral thymic factors remains hypothetical.

9. The Role of the Thymus in Immunologic Deficiency Disorders in Man

Immune defects in so-called immunologic deficiency syndromes in man (IDS) are the consequences of true developmental disorders which sets them in marked contrast to deficiency states that have been artificially induced by the postnatal ablation of immunologically active organs. Developmental failure of a particular organ or cell line with immunologic potential not only expresses itself in a functional deficiency or in the absence of one or more types of immunoglobulins, but also in morphologically detectable defects.

Experiments involving surgical or hormonal bursectomy and/or thymectomy in birds led to the hypothesis that thymus and bursa represent central precursor pools for two separate immunologically competent cell lines; thymus-derived cells would be responsible for the development and maintenance of transplantation immunity while bursa-derived cells would establish the immunoglobulin- and antibody-producing system (WARNER and SZENBERG, 1964; COOPER et al., 1965).

The production of immunoglobulins in mammals does not appear to be markedly affected by neonatal thymectomy, however, the combination of neonatal thymectomy and appendectomy in rabbits reportedly caused impairment in the production of both circulating immunoglobulins and humoral antibody (COOPER et al., 1967). GOOD et al. (1967) formulated a hypothesis in which a dissociation in the development of immunologic competence similar to the situation in birds is postulated also for mammals; these authors believe that in mammals, at least some part of, the gut-associated components of the Peyer's patch lymphoid tissue and the appendix may be regarded as "bursa-equivalent". The substance of this hypothesis is presented in Fig. 7 a. Hypothetical stem cells at a non-specified time in ontogeny may migrate into the thymus anlage or into the gut wall. From both locations these cells would then, after a period of proliferation and differentiation, reach lymphoid organs where they colonize thymus-dependent and "bursa-equivalent-dependent" areas, respectively (PARROT et al., 1966; COOPER et al., 1967; DE SOUSA and PARROT, 1967). Thymus-derived cells would be responsible exclusively for expressions of cellular immunity, whereas bursa-

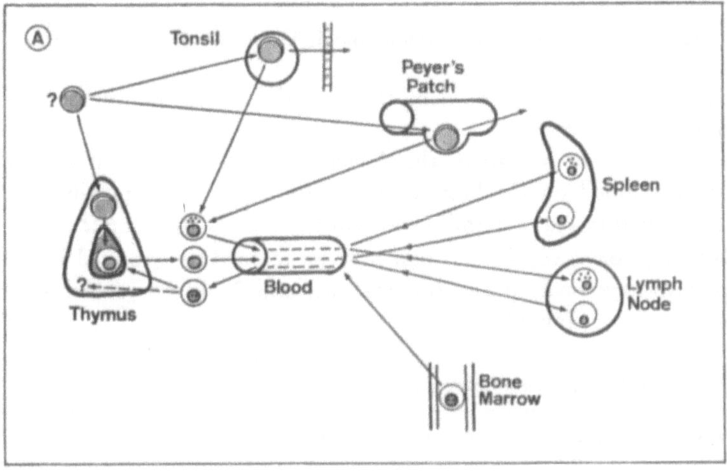

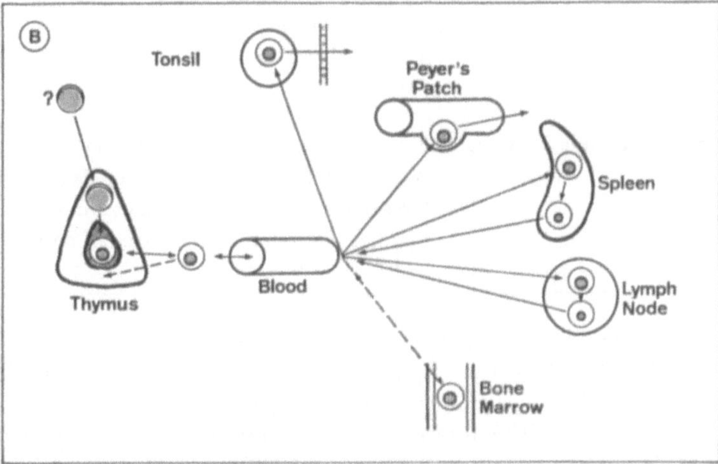

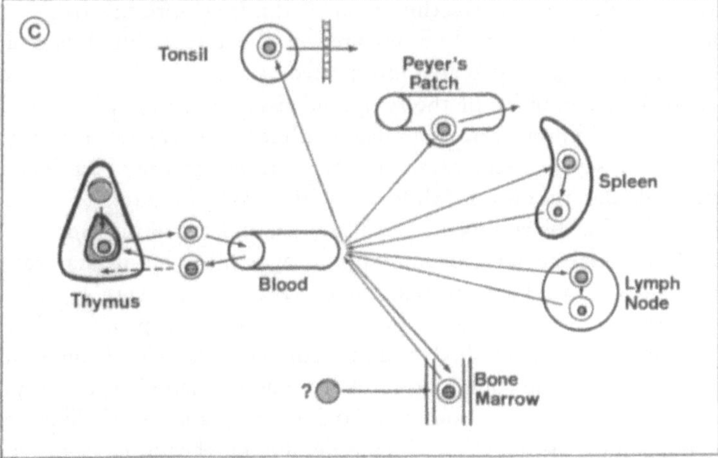

Fig. 7. Concepts of the origin of immunologically competent cells (see text pp. 70 ff.)
(cells leave the thymus via lymphatics)

equivalent-derived cells would be the exclusive source of immunoglobulins and humoral antibody.

As will be seen, not all of the defects observed in cases of IDS in man may be explained on the basis of this hypothesis; other possibilities have been illustrated in Fig. 7 b and c and will be referred to in the text.

Different forms of IDS in man may be tentatively grouped into 1. disorders with thymic dysplasia (or aplasia), and 2. disorders without severe thymic dysplasia (Table 10).

Table 10. *Immunologic deficiency syndromes (IDS) in man*

With thymic dysplasia (or aplasia)	Reticular dysgenesis
	Di George syndrome
	Swiss type agammaglobulinemia
	Thymic alymphoplasia
	(Ataxia-telangiectasia)
Without severe thymic dysplasia	BRUTON-type agammaglobulinemia
	Acquired forms of hypo- or agammaglobulinemia
	Dysgammaglobulinemia without lymphopenia
	Normogammaglobulinemic form of antibody deficiency disease

Several forms of IDS with developmental defects of the thymus have been described (see GOOD et al., 1967; COTTIER et al., 1967). Best defined among these various syndromes is the so-called *Swiss type of agammaglobulinemia* (SAG). The interpretation of this disease has changed considerably since GLANZMANN and RINIKER (1950) first observed the familial occurrence of deaths in early childhood of children suffering from extreme lymphopenia. The lack of lymphocytes in the circulating blood and in lymphoreticular organs was then interpreted as a massive loss of cells due to an increased vulnerability of the lymphoid tissue; it was not known at that time that these children were agammaglobulinemic. COTTIER (1957) was the first to show, seven years after the original observation, an incomplete descensus of the thymus in children with SAG; in addition, structural defects in the thymus rudiments were present, and a striking lack of plasma cells and germinal centers concomitant to agammaglobulinemia was noted in lymphoid organs. Patients with SAG suffer from severe lymphopenia, already present at the time of birth, an inability to produce detectable amounts of immunoglobulins, and a complete absence of humoral *and* cellular immunity. The combination of these defects led COTTIER to propose a developmental failure of both cellular immunity and of cell lines engaged in immunoglobulin production. A considerable number of cases of SAG has been described since 1950 (TOBLER and COTTIER, 1958; HITZIG et al., 1958; BARANDUN et al., 1959; HITZIG and WILLI, 1961).

The hypothesis that in mammals there may exist two separate cell lines of lymphoid cells, one derived from the thymus and the other from the "bursa-equivalent", is put to a severe test since in SAG both of these hypothetical cell lines are affected. If in the development of immunological competence lymphoid cells do originate from transformed thymic epithelial cells (AUERBACH, 1964 a), and if the precursors for immunoglobulin-producing cells stem from outside the thymus, then separate developmental defects of both systems would have to be postulated. If, however, these two systems have a common precursor cell at some time in early ontogenesis, the possibility of a single defect could be considered (GOOD et al., 1967). But this latter possibility would imply that either 1. not all of the thymic lymphoid cells originate from transformed epithelial cells (Fig. 7 b), or 2. thymus-derived lymphoid cells may also serve as precursors for the antibody-forming cell system (Fig. 7 c). In addition, it should be emphasized that the fact of the incomplete descensus of the thymus in SAG may hardly be explained by an extrathymic developmental defect.

Among the other syndromes of IDS with thymic defects, *thymic alymphoplasia* (ROSEN et al., 1962; GITLIN et al., 1964) most closely resembles SAG. In the few families in which thymic alymphoplasia was observed, only boys were affected. It may be possible that thymic alymphoplasia follows a sex-linked recessive inheritance, in contrast to SAG which is an autosomal recessive trait. The existence of two hereditary forms of IDS, one autosomal and one sex-linked, with almost identical structural and functional defects, is unexpected. According to the available reports, an incomplete descensus of the thymus may also be observed in cases with thymic alymphoplasia; both the degree of thymic structural defects and the degree of peripheral lymphopenia appear to be less pronounced than in cases with SAG. A distinction of the two forms of IDS on examination of histological preparations alone is very difficult if not impossible (COTTIER et al., 1967).

Mention should be made of a case of IDS with thymic structural defects reported by NEZELOF et al. (1964). In this particular case, the thymus was found to be very small although it had completed its descensus. An important difference between cases of SAG or thymic alymphoplasia on the one hand, and of NEZELOF's case on the other hand, lies in the fact that NEZELOF's patient had almost normal concentrations of circulating immunoglobulins. This particular situation has been compared to the combined effects of thymectomy and whole-body irradiation in birds, and has been cited as an example of "selective thymic developmental failure", in contrast to "development failure of the bursa-equivalent" (GOOD et al., 1967). However, NEZELOF et al., in the original publication, described an extremely rudimentary development of the gut-associated lymphoid structures. It is, therefore, rather difficult to prove normal development of the "bursa-equivalent".

Among less extensively studied forms of IDS with thymic defects, the *Di George syndrome* (DI GEORGE, 1965, 1967), also known under the "*III and IV Pharyngeal Pouch Syndrome*" (TAITZ et al., 1966), should be mentioned first. It is presently assumed that the disease may be caused by a combined developmental defect of the thymus and of the parathyroid; the consequences of this severe anlagen defect are difficult to assess and, since only a few cases have been described, adequate studies are not completed at the present time. It is of great importance to know whether the thymus in these cases is really absent or whether it may be found as a nondescended rudiment.

Ataxia-telangiectasia (or *Louis-Bar-Syndrome*) represents another example of a combined developmental defect: in addition to lesions located in the central nervous system, structural changes in the thymus have been reported in several cases (THIEFFRY et al., 1961; PETERSON et al., 1964). Again, an interpretation is difficult because of the superposition of consequences from the two defect systems; lymphopenia in these cases usually was less marked than in SAG or thymic alymphoplasia.

Reservations similar to those mentioned under SAG as to the justification of contrasting thymus-dependent and "bursa-equivalent"-dependent developmental failures may be made by examining reports on these forms of IDS. The presence of plasma cells has been described in cases of ataxia-telangiectasia, Di George syndrome (DI GEORGE, 1965; TAITZ et al., 1966) and in other forms of thymic alymphoplasia in combination with the formation of germinal centers without (MATSANIOTIS et al., 1966) or with the presence of circulating immunoglobulins (FULGINITI et al., 1966) or dys-gammaglobulinemia (BRETON et al., 1963; FIREMAN et al., 1966). As has been stressed by KADOWAKI et al. (1965), HARBOE et al. (1966), and COTTIER et al. (1967), it is of great importance to know whether the plasma cells in these cases are the patient's own elements or whether they derive from a successful graft, be it from the mother, from transfusions of fresh blood, or from transplants. As long as a chimerism of this kind has not been excluded by testing the genetically determined properties of cells and their products, a final evaluation of these cases may not be possible. Only if a transfer of immunologically competent cells from a healthy individual to the afflicted child can be excluded, these particular forms of IDS would present a strong case in favor of the existence of two separate systems in the development of immunological competence.

In the group of diseases without severe thymic dysplasia the best known and the most extensively studied form of IDS is the *classical, sex-linked agammaglobulinemia* (BRUTON, 1952). The inability of patients with

Bruton's agammaglobulinemia to produce immunoglobulin in appreciable concentrations is reflected morphologically in an extreme scarcity of plasma cells and germinal centers, even after repeated antigenic stimulation; the defect may, however, not be absolute in many cases. Lymphoid tissue in the gut wall, in tonsils, in spleen or in lymph nodes is present in considerable amounts; no evidence was found for a distinct arrangement of lymphoid cells in zones of spleen and lymph nodes (COTTIER et al., 1967) equivalent to the "thymus-dependent" areas in mice (PARROT et al., 1966; DE SOUSA and PARROT, 1967). It is not known whether the hypothetical stem cells which may represent precursors for all antibody-forming cells are absent, or whether they are present but cannot transform into germinal center cells or plasma cells due to some unknown genetically determined defect. It is of interest to note that in a number of cases of *Bruton's* agammaglobulinemia considerably prolonged rejection times for skin homografst were also observed (BARANDUN et al., 1959). Evidently more data are needed to exclude some degree of thymic failure combined with the defect of the immunoglobulin-producing system.

Other types of diseases with defective immunoglobulin production are still ill-defined entities. They have been discussed by GOOD et al. (1967), COTTIER et al. (1967) and STOELINGA (1966).

Study of these different forms of developmental immunopathies appears to be of critical importance since it may be the only feasible way to obtain more precise knowledge on the ontogenetic development and specific physiological function(s) of different types of immunoglobulins and of different cell types involved in immune reactions.

10. Conclusions

In reviewing the presently available data, progress that has been made during the last few years towards a better understanding of the role(s) of the thymus may be summarized as follows.

Phylogenetic studies revealed that the capacity to respond to various kinds of antigenic stimulation developed together with the step-wise deployment of first a lympho-myeloid complex (cyclostomes), then thymus and spleen (lower elasmobranchs), then plasma cells (higher elasmobranchs, chondrostean and teleost fish), then lymph nodes (some amphibians, reptiles), then germinal centers and tonsils (birds, reptiles, mammals). The analogy between phylogenetic and ontogenetic development of the lympho-reticular system is only partial; it may be noted that, among other incongruencies, in man as well as in other mammals lymph nodes are formed well before the first plasma cells appear, a sequence of events which is in contrast to that observed in phylogenetic studies.

There is general agreement that during ontogenesis of most mammalian species the thymus is the first organ to contain numerous lymphoid cells. The origin of these cells, however, is still disputed. If AUERBACH's interpretation of his *in vitro* experiments is correct, and if it may be extrapolated to *in vivo* conditions, we must assume that most if not all thymic lymphoid cells during early embryogenesis originate in the thymus itself (Fig. 7 c). Since it has been repeatedly shown that under certain experimental conditions lymphoid cells, especially those from the bone marrow, may enter the thymus of the adult animal, it may have to be assumed that in postnatal life part of the lymphoid population of the thymus is constantly being exchanged by immigrating cells.

These immigrating cells supposedly are primitive (often called "noncommitted", immature, or incompetent) cells which, according to the prevailing hypothesis, would be transformed in the thymus into cells with the potential to react to antigenic stimulation. Studies showed that the more primitive cells in the thymus are located in the cortex; in the course of their differentiation and maturation they shift to the medulla from where they eventually leave the organ or where they die under the influence of some unknown regulatory mechanism. It is not known how cells may migrate from a distant site to enter the thymus in a "virginal" state; for want of a better explanation a dedifferentiation process has been proposed to take place in the thymic cortex. These mechanisms are still poorly understood, and there is great need for more detailed studies on both kinetics of thymic cells and the immunological potential of cortical *versus* medullary thymic lymphocytes.

A correlation between the degree of lymphoid development and the ability to perform immune functions during ontogenesis has been revealed in studies which indicate that antibody formation or skin graft rejection occur only when the thymus has assumed its lymphoid appearance and when circulating lymphocytes are present in the peripheral blood. SILVERSTEIN's investigations on immunological capacities of fetal lambs show that responsiveness to some antigens may be acquired earlier than that to others (SILVERSTEIN, 1964; SILVERSTEIN and KRANER, 1965).

In view of these findings on the ontogeny of the capacity to respond to antigenic stimulation it is not surprising that neonatal thymectomy would have such a variable effect on immune functions. Even when performed immediately after birth, thymectomy may be too late to prevent the establishment of a certain degree of immune responsiveness to stimulation with some antigens. Even intrauterine thymectomy in fetal lambs was largely ineffective in interfering with the development of antibody-forming capacity to certain antigens (SILVERSTEIN and KRANER, 1965). No experimental data exist which indicate the approximative time of the first thymic influence on the development of immunity in ontogeny. The development of methods for intrauterine experimentation would greatly enhance the propects of widening understanding of the role of the thymus in the ontogenetic development of the lympho-reticular system and of immune responsiveness.

A comparison of the varied effects of thymectomy appears to be almost futile in view of the diversified experimental conditions and methods used to assess the immunological capacity of the thymectomized animal. The occurrence of wasting disease in thymectomized, conventionally raised animals, even when clinically not apparent, drastically obscures the results obtained. As long as animal strains other than pathogen- or germfree are used in thymectomy studies, the true effects of thymus deprivation on both the lympho-reticular structures and cells, and on immune responsiveness may not be clearly discerned.

Although the question of the etiology of post-thymectomy wasting has not been resolved, overwhelming evidence points to systemic infection as the origin of the disease. The infectious agents involved have not been specified so far; presumably they may represent the normal bacterial flora of the animal. It would not be surprising if antibody-activity against these unknown organisms and pathogens were eventually demonstrated in the serum of wasting, thymectomized animals. An alternative and less than plausible explanation of the very irregularly increased production of some immunoglobulins in animals suffering from wasting would be the expression of an uncontrolled gammaglobulin turnout resulting in the formation of "nonsense"-immunoglobulins (COOPER et al., 1967).

Even if neonatal thymectomy, or adult thymectomy in combination with whole-body irradiation, is not followed by complete abolishment of immune responsiveness, and, therefore, may not be the ideal immunosuppressive therapy as it was originally thought, thymectomized animals can serve as valuable aids in studies designed to learn more about the mechanisms involved in certain immune reactions. For example, thymectomy causes a marked impairment of anamnestic antibody responses in some animals to certain antigens and a marked delay in homograft rejection; this presents an unresolved dilemma since anamnestic responses are most difficult to suppress by any other means.

Severe or complete developmental failure of the thymus and its dependent cells, in some forms of immunological deficiency diseases in man, presents a picture quite different from the one encountered in experimentally thymectomized animals. As has been discussed in the preceeding chapter, the convenient hypothesis of a separation into thymus- and "bursa-equivalent"-dependent cell lines in man raises many questions. Until the time that the current inconsistencies between theoretical expectation and clinical finding have been satisfyingly resolved, the separation in man of the lympho-reticular system into the progeny of two different cell populations appears to be speculative.

Thus, the cardinal role(s) of the thymus still remain obscure. Research on the functions of the thymus has passed through another peak of great excitement and world-wide activity. A few facts, however, have emerged and are deemed worthy of reemphasis. It appears undeniable that the thymus plays an important if not decisive part in the initial establishment of potential immunological competence during early ontogenesis of the mammalian organism. Most likely the thymus acts directly by supplying lymphoid cells to other lymphoid tissues. The origin of these lymphoid cells is still disputed; in early embryogenesis they may have their origin exclusively in the thymus itself, in later life they may, at least in part, represent the progeny of cells that immigrated the thymus. Export of lymphoid cells from the thymus continues throughout life; the rate at which these cells leave the thymus may be subject to several regulatory mechanisms (hormonal influences, stress, immunological requirements etc.).

Convincing evidence for other thymic functions, such as the production of humoral and/or contact factors for control of lymphoid proliferation and differentiation in embryogenesis and in adult life, the elimination of clones of cells with anti-"self" reactivity, and the production of trephocytic substances, is still lacking or inconclusive. Until these various substances are isolated in a biologically active form, and until it can be demonstrated that, instead of being only one target organ among many, the thymus also plays an active role in control of autoimmune processes, these humoral aspects of thymic function remain hypothetical conceptions.

Literature

ACKERMAN, G. A.: Electron microscopy of the bursa of Fabricius of the embryonic chick with particular reference to the lympho-epithelial nodules. J. cell. Biol. **13**, 127—146 (1962).

—, and R. A. KNOUFF: Lymphocytopoiesis in the bursa of Fabricius. Amer. J. Anat. **104**, 163—205 (1959).

— — Lymphocyte formation in the thymus of the embryonic chick. Anat. Rec. **149**, 191—216 (1964).

ADA, G. L., G. J. V. NOSSAL, and J. PYE: Antigens in immunity. XI. The uptake of antigen in animals previously rendered immunologically tolerant. Aust. J. exp. biol. med. Sci. **43**, 337—344 (1965).

ADNER, M. M., J. D. SHERMAN, and W. DAMESHEK: The normal development of the lymphoid mass in the golden hamster and its relationship to the effects of thymectomy. Blood **25**, 511—521 (1965).

AISENBERG, A. C., B. WILKES, and B. H. WAKSMAN: The production of runt disease in rats thymectomized at birth. J. exp. Med. **116**, 759—772 (1962).

— — Partial restoration of neonatally thymectomized rats with thymus-containing diffusion chambers. Nature (Lond.) **205**, 716—717 (1965).

ALBRIGHT, J. F., and T. MAKINODAN: Dynamics of expression of competence of antibody-producing cells. In: Molecular and cellular basis of antibody formation (J. STERZL, ed.). Prague-New York-London: Academic Press 1965, pp. 427—446.

ALLIBONE, E. C., W. GOLDIE, and B. P. MARMION: *Pneumocystis carinii* pneumonia and progressive vaccinia in siblings. Arch. Dis. Childh. **39**, 26—34 (1964).

ANDERSEN, D. H.: The relationship between the thymus and reproduction. Physiol. Rev. **12**, 1—22 (1932).

ANDREASEN, E., and J. OTTESEN: Significance of the various lymphoid organs to the lymphocyte production in the albino rat. Acta path. microbiol. scand. **54**, 25—32 (1944).

— — Studies on the lymphocyte production. Investigations on the nucleic acid turnover in the lymphoid organs. Acta physiol. scand. **10**, 258—270 (1945).

—, and S. CHRISTENSEN: The rate of mitotic activity in the lymphoid organs of the rat. Anat. Rec. **103**, 401—412 (1949).

ARCHER, O. K., and J. C. PIERCE: Role of the thymus in development of the immune response. Fed. Proc. **20**, 26 (1961) (Abstract).

— —, B. W. PAPERMASTER, and R. A. GOOD: Reduced antibody response in thymectomized rabbits. Nature (Lond.) **195**, 191—192 (1962).

—, D. E. R. SUTHERLAND, and R. A. GOOD: The developmental biology of lymphoid tissue in the rabbit. Consideration of the role of thymus and appendix. Lab. Invest. **13**, 259—271 (1964 a).

—, B. W. PAPERMASTER, and R. A. GOOD: Thymectomy in rabbit and mouse: Consideration of time of lymphoid peripheralization. In: The thymus in immunobiology (R. A. GOOD and A. E. GABRIELSEN, eds.). New York: Hoeber-Harper 1964 b, pp. 414—431.

ARGYRIS, B. F.: Effect of thymus grafts, spleen cell injection and sublethal irradiation on homograft tolerance in mice. Transplantation **3**, 350—355 (1965).

ARNASON, B. G., and B. D. JANKOVIC: Suppression of "delayed" hypersensitivity reactions in rats thymectomized at birth. Fed. Proc. **21**, 274 (1962) (Abstract).

— —, and B. H. WAKSMAN: A survey of the thymus and its relation to lymphocytes and immune reactions. Blood **20**, 617—628 (1962 a).

— — —, and C. WENNERSTEN: Role of the thymus in immune reactions in rats. II. Suppressive effect of thymectomy at birth in reactions of delayed (cellular) hypersensitivity and the circulating small lymphocyte. J. exp. Med. **116**, 177—186 (1962 b).

— — — Effect of thymectomy on "delayed" hypersensitivity reactions. Nature (Lond.) **194**, 99—100 (1962 c).

—, C. DE VAUX ST. CYR, and J. B. SHAFFNER: A comparison of immunoglobulins and antibody production in the normal and thymectomized mouse. J. Immunol. **93**, 915—925 (1964 a).

—, B. D. JANKOVIC, and B. H. WAKSMAN: The role of the thymus in immune reactions in rats. In: The thymus in immunobiology (R. A. GOOD, and A. E. GABRIELSEN, eds.). New York: Hoeber-Harper 1964 b, pp. 492—501.

—, C. DE VAUX ST. CYR, and E. H. RELYFELD: Role of the thymus in immune reactions in rats. IV. Immunoglobulins and antibody formation. Int. Arch. Allergy **25**, 206—224 (1964 c).

ASPINALL, R. L., R. K. MEYER, M. A. GRAETZER, and H. R. WOLFE: Effect of thymectomy and bursectomy on the survival of skin homografts in chickens. J. Immunol. **90**, 872—877 (1963).

AUERBACH, R.: Morphogenetic interactions in the development of the mouse thymus gland. Develop. Biol. **2**, 271—284 (1960).

— Experimental analysis of the origin of cell types in the development of the mouse thymus. Develop. Biol. **3**, 336—354 (1961 a).

— Genetic control of thymus lymphoid differentiation. Proc. nat. Acad. Sci. (USA) **47**, 1175—1181 (1961 b).

AUERBACH, R.: Developmental studies of mouse thymus and spleen. J. nat. Cancer Inst. 11, 23—33 (1963).
— Experimental analysis of mouse thymus and spleen morphogenesis. In: The thymus in immunobiology (R. A. GOOD and A. E. GABRIELSEN, eds.). New York: Hoeber-Harper 1964 a, pp. 95—113.
— On the function of the embryonic thymus. In: The thymus (V. DEFENDI and D. METCALF, eds.). Philadelphia: The Wistar Institute Press 1964 b, pp. 1—7.
— Embryogenesis of immune systems. In: Thymus. Experimental and clinical studies (G. E. W. WOLSTENHOLME and R. PORTER, eds.). London: Churchill 1966, pp. 39—49.
AXELRAD, A. A., and H. C. VAN DER GAAG: Susceptibility to lymphoma induction by Gross' passage A virus in C3Hf/Bi mice of different ages: Relation to thymic cell multiplication and differentiation. J. nat. Cancer Inst. 28, 1065—1093 (1962).
AZAR, H. A., G. NAUJOK, and J. WILLIAMS: Role of the adult thymus in immune reactions. I. Observations on lymphoid organs, circulating lymphocytes and serum protein fractions of thymectomized or splenectomized adult mice. Amer. J. Path. 43, 213—225 (1963).
—, J. WILLIAMS, and K. TAKATSUKI: Development of plasma cells and immunoglobulins in neonatally thymectomized rats. In: The thymus (V. DEFENDI and D. METCALF, eds.). Philadelphia: The Wistar Institute Press 1964, pp. 75—87.
BADERTSCHER, J. A.: The development of the thymus in the pig. II. Histogenesis. Amer. J. Anat. 17, 437—493 (1915).
BAER, J. G.: Immunité et réactions immunitaires chez les invertébrés. Schweiz. Z. allg. Path. Bakt. 7, 442—462 (1944).
BAERLOCHER, K., F. BALMER u. U. KRECH: Der klinische und virologische Verlauf einer konnatalen Rubellainfektion. Schweiz. med. Wschr. 97, 904—911 (1967).
BALL, W. D., and R. AUERBACH: *In vitro* formation of lymphocytes from embryonic thymus. Exp. Cell Res. 20, 245—247 (1960).
— A quantitative assessment of mouse thymus differentiation. Exp. Cell Res. 31, 82—88 (1963).
BALNER, H., and H. DERSJANT: Sex difference for immune depression and runting in neonatally thymectomized mice. Nature (Lond.) 209, 815—816 (1966).
BANGHAM, D. R., P. M. COTES, K. R. HOBBS, and D. E. H. TEE: An attempt to determine the age at which "cellular immunological maturity" develops in the foetal rhesus monkey. In: Proc. Intern. Symp. "Bone Marrow Therapy and Chemical Protection in Irradiated Primates". Rijswijk: Radiobiological Institute TNO 1962, pp. 187—194.
BARANDUN, S., H. COTTIER, A. HÄSSIG u. G. RIVA (eds.): Das Antikörpermangelsyndrom. Basel-Stuttgart: Benno Schwabe 1959.
BARCLAY, T. J., I. L. WEISSMAN, and H. S. KAPLAN: Discussion remark. In: The thymus (V. DEFENDI and D. METCALF, eds.). Philadelphia: The Wistar Institute Press 1964, pp. 117—119.
BARNES, D. W. H., J. F. LOUTIT, and J. M. SANSOM: Role of the thymus in the radiation chimera. Ann. N. Y. Acad. Sci. 120, 218—224 (1964).
BART, R. S., R. STRITZLER, and R. L. BAER: Failure of thymectomy in newborn guinea pigs to influence contact sensitization to dinitrochlorobenzene. J. Immunol. 97, 477—483 (1966).
BASCH, R. S.: Immunologic competence after thymectomy. Int. Arch. Allergy 30, 105—119 (1966).
BAZIN, H., et J. F. DUPLAN: Modifications du taux des immunoglobulines chez des souris thymectomisées à l'âge adulte et irradiées. Rev. franç. Et. clin. biol. 11, 987—1000 (1967).

BEALMEAR, P. M., and R. WILSON: Homograft rejection by neonatally thymectomized germ-free mice. Cancer Res. **27**, 358—361 (1967 a).
— — Personal communication (1967 b).
BEARD, J.: The development and probable function of the thymus. Anat. Anz. **9**, 476—486 (1895).
— The source of leucocytes and the true function of the thymus. Anat. Anz. **18**, 550—573 (1900).
BIERRING, F.: Quantitative investigations on the lymphomyeloid system in thymectomized rats. In: Haemopoiesis; cell production and its regulation (G. E. W. WOLSTENHOLME and M. O'CONNOR, eds.). Boston: Churchill; Little, Brown 1960, pp. 185—198.
BIGGART, J. D.: The influence of thymus grafts in diffusion chambers on the lymphoid tissues of neonatally thymectomized rats. Brit. J. exp. Path. **47**, 586—589 (1966 a).
— The influence of thymus grafts in diffusion chambers on the immunological system of neonatally thymectomized rats. Brit. J. exp. Path. **47**, 590—593 (1966 b).
BISSET, K. A.: Bacterial infection and immunity in lower vertebrates and invertebrates. J. Hyg. **45**, 128—135 (1947).
BLOCK, M.: The blood forming tissues and blood of the newborn opossum *(Didelphys Virginiana)*. I. Normal development through about the one hundreth day of life. Erg. Anat. Entwickl.-Gesch. **37**, 237—366 (1964).
BRETON, A., R. WALBAUM, L. BONIFACE, M. GOUDEMAND et A. DUPONT: Lymphocytophthisie avec dysgammaglobulinémie chez un nourrisson. Arch. franç. Pédiat. **20**, 131—146 (1963).
BROOKE, M. S.: The immunological behaviour of mature C57BL/6J mice thymectomized ad birth. Immunology **8**, 526—528 (1965).
BRUMBY, M., and D. METCALF: Migration of cells to the thymus demonstrated by parabiosis. Proc. Soc. exp. Biol. Med. **124**, 99—103 (1967).
BRUTON, O. C.: Agammaglobulinemia. Pediatrics **9**, 722—728 (1952).
BURNET, F. M.: Immunological recognition of self. Science **133**, 307—311 (1961).
— Role of the thymus and related organs in immunity. Brit. med. J. **2**, 807—811 (1962).
CALNE, R. Y.: Thymectomy in dogs with renal homografts treated with drugs. Nature (Lond.) **199**, 388—389 (1963).
CAMBLIN, J. G., and J. B. BRIDGES: Effects of cell-free extracts of thymus in leucopenic rats. Transplantation **2**, 785—787 (1964).
CAMERON, G. R.: Inflammation in earthworms. J. Path. Bact. **35**, 933—972 (1932).
— Inflammation in the caterpillars of *Lepidoptera*. J. Path. Bact. **38**, 441—466 (1934).
CAMPBELL, D. H., and J. S. GARVEY: Nature of retained antigen and its role in immune mechanisms. Adv. Immunol. **3**, 261—313 (1963).
CANTACUZÈNE, J.: Le problème de l'immunité chez les invertébrés. Paris: Masson 1923.
CAREY, J., and N. L. WARNER: Gamma-globulin synthesis in hormonally bursectomized chickens. Nature (Lond.) **203**, 198—199 (1964).
CHANG, T. S., B. GLICK, and A. R. WINTER: The significance of the bursa of Fabricius of chickens in antibody production. Poultry Sci. **34**, 1187 (1955) (Abstract).
CLAFLIN, A. J., O. SMITHIES, and R. K. MEYER: Antibody responses in bursa-deficient chickens. J. Immunol. **97**, 693—699 (1966).
CLAMAN, H. N., and D. W. TALMAGE: Thymectomy: Prolongation of immunological tolerance in the adult mouse. Science **141**, 1193—1194 (1963).
—, and W. McDONALD: Thymus and X-radiation in the termination of acquired immunological tolerance in the adult mouse. Nature (Lond.) **202**, 712—713 (1964).

CLARK, S. L.: Cytological evidences of secretion in the thymus. In: Thymus. Experimental and clinical studies (G. E. W. WOLSTENHOLME and R. PORTER, eds.). London: Churchill 1966, pp. 3—30.

COMSA, C.: Consequences of thymectomy upon the leucopoiesis in guinea pigs. Acta endocrin. **26**, 361—365 (1957).

— Action of the purified thymus hormone in thymectomized guinea pigs. Amer. J. med. Sci. **250**, 79—85 (1965).

COOPER, E. L., and W. H. HILDEMANN: Allograft rejection in bullfrog larvae in relation to thymectomy. Transplantation **3**, 446—448 (1965).

COOPER, M. D., R. D. A. PETERSON, and R. A. GOOD: Delineation of the thymic and bursal lymphoid systems in the chicken. Nature (Lond.) **205**, 143—146 (1965).

— —, M. A. SOUTH, and R. A. GOOD: The functions of the thymus system and the bursa system in the chickens. J. exp. Med. **123**, 75—102 (1966 a).

—, M. L. SCHWARTZ, and R. A. GOOD: Restoration of gamma globulin production in agammaglobulinemic chickens. Science **151**, 471—473 (1966 b).

—, D. Y. PEREY, M. F. McKNEALLY, A. E. GABRIELSEN, D. E. R. SUTHERLAND, and R. A. GOOD: A mammalian equivalent of the avian bursa of Fabricius. Lancet **1**, 1388—1391 (1966 a).

—, A. E. GABRIELSEN, R. D. A. PETERSON, and R. A. GOOD: Ontogenetic development of the germinal centers and their function — relationship to the bursa of Fabricius. In: Germinal centers in immune responses (H. COTTIER, N. ODARTCHENKO, R. SCHINDLER, and C. C. CONGDON, eds.). Berlin-Heidelberg-New York: Springer 1967, pp. 28—33.

CORSI, A., and G. V. GIUSTI: Phagocytic activity after thymectomy. Nature (Lond.) **213**, 618—619 (1967).

COTTIER, H.: Zur Histopathologie des Antikörpermangelsyndroms. Trans. 6th Congr. Europ. Soc. Haemat., Copenhagen, 1957. Basel-New York: Karger 1958, pp. 41 —46.

— Strahlenbedingte Lebensverkürzung. Berlin-Göttingen-Heidelberg: Springer 1961.

—, N. ODARTCHENKO, G. KEISER, M. HESS, and R. D. STONER: Incorporation of tritiated nucleosides and amino acids into lymphoid and plasmocytoid cells during secondary response to tetanus toxoid in mice. Ann. N. Y. Acad. Sci. **113**, 612—626 (1964 a).

— —, L. E. FEINENDEGEN, and V. P. BOND: Tritiated thymidine for *in vivo* cytokinetic studies on lymphoreticular tissue. In: The thymus in immunobiology (R. A. GOOD and A. E. GABRIELSEN, eds.). New York: Hoeber-Harper 1964 b, pp. 332—340.

— Etudes de cinétique cellulaire effectuées sur des thymus "Swiss albino" au cours de la période périnatale en utilisant, comme indicateur, une substance marquée, la thymidine-³H. Méd. Hyg. **23**, 794 (1965).

— Studi citocinetici sul timo di topi albini Swiss nel periodo perinatale mediante timidina-³H. In: Atti del Convegno sul Timo, Cernobbio, 1965. Minerva ped. (Torino) 1966, pp. 9—11.

—, G. KEISER, N. ODARTCHENKO, M. HESS, and R. D. STONER: *De novo* formation and rapid growth of germinal centers during secondary antibody responses to tetanus toxoid in mice. In: Germinal centers in immune responses (H. COTTIER, N. ODARTCHENKO, R. SCHINDLER, and C. C. CONGDON, eds.). Berlin-Heidelberg-New York: Springer 1967, pp. 270—276.

—, K. BÜRKI, M. W. HESS, and A. HÄSSIG: Pathologic considerations of immunologic deficiency diseases in man. In: Proc. 3rd Developmental Immunology Workshop, Florida (1967) (in press).

CRADDOCK, C. G., G. S. NAKAI, H. FUKUTA, and L. M. VANSLAGER: Proliferative activity of the lymphatic tissues of rats as studied with tritium-labeled thymidine. J. exp. Med. 120, 389—412 (1964).

CRONKITE, E. P.: Discussion remark. In: Germinal centers in immune responses (H. COTTIER, N. ODARTCHENKO, R. SCHINDLER, and C. C. CONGDON, eds.). Berlin-Heidelberg-New York: Springer 1967, pp. 166—167.

CROSS, A. M., E. LEUCHARS, and J. F. A. P. MILLER: Studies on the recovery of the immune response in irradiated mice thymectomized in adult life. J. exp. Med. 119, 837—850 (1964).

DALMASSO, A. P., C. MARTINEZ, and R. A. GOOD: Failure of spleen cells from thymectomized mice to induce graft *vs.* host reactions. Proc. Soc. exp. Biol. Med. 110, 205—208 (1962).

DALMASSO, A. P., C. MARTINEZ, K. SJODIN, and R. A. GOOD: Studies on the role of the thymus in immunobiology. Reconstitution of immunologic capacity in mice thymectomized at birth. J. exp. Med. 118, 1089—1109 (1963).

DAMESHEK, W.: The thymus and lymphoid proliferation. Blood 20, 629—632 (1962).

DAVIS, W. E., JR., M. L. TYAN, and L. J. COLE: Homografts in thymectomized, irradiated mice: Responses to primary and secondary skin grafts. Science 145, 394—395 (1964).

DEFENDI, V., and D. METCALF (eds.): The thymus (Symposium held at the Wistar Institute of Anatomy and Biology, Philadelphia, 1964). Philadelphia: The Wistar Institute Press 1964.

—, R. A. ROOSA, and H. KOPROWSKI: Effect of thymectomy at birth on response to tissue, cells and virus antigen. In: The thymus in immunobiology (R. A. GOOD and A. E. GABRIELSEN, eds.). New York: Hoeber-Harper 1964, pp. 504—521.

DE SOMER, P., P. DENYS, JR., and R. LEYTEN: Activity of a non-cellular calf thymus extract in normal and thymectomized mice. Life Sci. 11, 810—819 (1963).

DE SOUSA, M. A. B., and D. M. V. PARROT: The definition of a germinal center area as distinct from the thymus-dependent area in the lymphoid tissue of the mouse. In: Germinal centers in immune responses (H. COTTIER, N. ODARTCHENKO, R. SCHINDLER and C. C. CONGDON, eds.). Berlin-Heidelberg-New York: Springer 1967, pp. 361—370.

DE VRIES, M. J., L. M. VAN PUTTEN, H. BALNER, and D. W. VAN BEKKUM: Lésions suggérant une réactivité auto-immune chez des souris thymectomisées à la naissance. Rev. franç. Et. clin. biol. 9, 381—397 (1964).

— Discussion remark. Proc. 3rd Immunol. Dev. Workshop, Florida 1967 (in press).

DE WINIWATER, H.: Recherches sur l'évolution des dérivés branchiaux et l'histogénèse du thymus (cobaye). Arch. Biol. 44, 741—808 (1933).

DIDERHOLM, H., and K. E. FICHTELIUS: An autoradiographic study of the difference between thymus and lymph node lymphocytes shown by transfusion of labelled cells. Acta haemat. 22, 112—117 (1959).

— Studies on the migration and transformation of lymphocytes in immunized and nonimmunized animals. Acta path. microbiol. scand. Suppl. 146 (1961).

DIENER, E., and E. H. M. EALEY: Immune system in a monotreme: Studies on the Australian echidna *(Tachyglossus aculeatus)*. Nature (Lond.) 208, 950—953 (1965).

DI GEORGE, A. M.: Discussion of a paper by M. D. COOPER et al. J. Pediat. 67, 907 (1965).

— Congenital absence of the human thymus and its immunologic consequences. In: Proc. 3rd Developmental Immunology Workshop, Florida (1967) (in press).

DOUGHERTY, T. F.: Effect of hormones on lymphatic tissue. Physiol. Rev. 32, 379—401 (1952).

DREYER, N. B., and J. W. KING: Anaphylaxis in the fish. J. Immunol. 60, 277—282 (1948).

DUKOR, P., and F. M. DIETRICH: Chemical suppression of immune responses in thymectomized mice. Int. Arch. Allergy 32, 131—148 (1967).

—, J. F. A. P. MILLER, W. HOUSE, and V. ALLMAN: Regeneration of thymus grafts. I. Histological and cytological aspects. Transplantation 3, 639—668 (1965).

—, F. M. DIETRICH, and M. ROSENTHAL: Recovery of immunological responsiveness in thymectomized mice. Clin. exp. Immunol. 1, 391—404 (1966).

DU PASQUIER, L.: Aspects cellulaires et humoraux de l'intolérance aux homogreffes de tissue musculaire chez le têtard d' *Alytes obstetricans:* rôle du thymus. C. R. Soc. Biol. 261, 1144—1147 (1965).

DUSTIN, A. P.: Recherches d'histologie normale et expérimentale sur le thymus des amphibiens anoures. 1ère partie: Structure normale, variations saisonnières, variations expérimentales. Arch. Biol. 28, 1—110 (1913).

EAST, J., D. M. V. PARROT, F. C. CHESTERMAN, and A. POMERANCE: The appearance of a hepatotrophic virus in mice thymectomized at birth. J. exp. Med. 118, 1069—1082 (1963).

EICHENWALD, H. F., and H. R. SHINEFELD: Antibody production by the human fetus. J. Pediat. 63, 870 (1963).

EISEN, N. H., and F. KARUSH: Immune tolerance and an extracellular regulatory role for bivalent antibody. Nature (Lond.) 202, 677—682 (1964).

ERNSTRÖM, U., L. GYLLENSTEN, and B. LARSSON: Venous output of lymphocytes from the thymus. Nature (Lond.) 207, 540—541 (1965).

—, and B. LARSSON: Thymic and thoracic duct contributions to blood lymphocytes in normal and thyroxin-treated guinea pigs. Acta physiol. scand. 66, 189—195 (1966).

EVERETT, N. B., W. O. RIEKE, and R. N. CAFFREY: The kinetics of small lymphocytes in the rat, with special reference to those of thymic origin. In: The thymus in immunobiology (R. A. GOOD and A. E. GABRIELSEN, ed.). New York: Hoeber-Harper 1964, pp. 291—297.

FAHEY, J. L., W. F. BARTH, and L. W. LAW: Normal immunoglobulins and antibody response in neonatally thymectomized mice. J. nat. Cancer Inst. 35, 663—678 (1965).

FELDMAN, M., and A. GLOBERSON: The role of the thymus in restoring immunological reactivity and lymphoid cell differentiation in X-irradiated adult mice. Ann. N. Y. Acad. Sci. 120, 182—190 (1964).

FELTON, L. D., G. KAUFFMANN, B. PRESCOTT, and B. OTTINGER: Studies on the mechanism of the immunological paralysis induced in mice by pneumococcal polysaccharides. J. Immunol. 74, 17—26 (1955).

FENNESTAD, K. L., and C. BORG-PETERSEN: Antibody formation in bovine foetuses infected with *Leptospira saxkoebing*. Acta path. microbiol. scand. Suppl. 154, 307—308 (1962).

FICHTELIUS, K. E.: A difference between lymph nodal and thymic lymphocytes shown by transfusion of labelled cells. Acta anat. 32, 114—125 (1958).

— On the destination of thymic lymphocytes. In: Haemopoiesis: Cell production and its regulation (G. E. W. WOLSTENHOLME and M. O'CONNOR, eds.). Boston: Churchill; Little, Brown 1960, pp. 204—220.

—, G. LAURELL, and L. PHILIPSSON: The influence of thymectomy on antibody formation. Acta path. microbiol. scand. 51, 81—86 (1961).

FINSTAD, J., and R. A. GOOD: Phylogenetic studies of adaptive immune responses in the lower vertebrates. In: Phylogeny of immunity (R. T. SMITH, P. A. MIESCHER and R. A. GOOD, eds.). Jacksonville: Univ. of Florida Press 1966, pp. 173—188.

FIREMAN, P., H. A. JOHNSON, and D. GITLIN: Plasma cells, γ_1M-Globulin in thymic alymphoplasia. Pediatrics 37, 485—492 (1966).

FISHER, B., E. R. FISHER, S. LEE, and A. SAKAI: Renal homotransplantation in neonatal thymectomized puppies. Transplantation 3, 49—53 (1965).

FISHER, E. R., and B. FISHER: Role of the thymus in skin and tumor transplantation in the rat. Lab. Invest. 14, 546—555 (1965).

FOLLET, D. A., J. R. BATTISTO, and B. R. BLOOM: Tolerance to a defined chemical hapten produced in adult guinea-pigs after thymectomy. Immunology 11, 73—76 (1966).

FORD, C. E.: Traffic of lymphoid cells in the body. In: Thymus. Experimental and clinic studies (G. E. W. WOLSTENHOLME and R. PORTER, eds.). London: Churchill 1966, pp. 131—152.

FORD, W. L., J. L. GOWANS, and P. J. McCULLAGH: The origin and function of lymphocytes. In: Thymus. Experimental and clinical studies (G. E. W. WOLSTENHOLME and R. PORTER, eds.). London: Churchill 1966, pp. 59—79.

FRIDRICH, R., and M. SCHÄFER: The influence of the thymus on radiogold clearance. Experientia 22, 552—553 (1966).

FRIEDMAN, H.: Absence of antibody plaque forming cells in spleens of thymectomized mice immunized with sheep erythrocytes. Proc. Soc. exp. Biol. Med. 118, 1176—1180 (1965).

FULGINITI, V. A., W. E. HATHAWAY, D. S. PEARLMAN, W. R. BLACKBURN, J. H. GITHENS, H. N. CLAMAN, and C. H. KEMPE: Dissociation of delayed hypersensitivity in man. Report of two sibships with thymic dysplasia, lymphoid tissue depletion, and normal immunoglobulins. Lancet 2, 5—8 (1966).

GABRIELSEN, A. E., and R. A. GOOD: Thymoma. Ann. int. Med. 65, 607—611 (1966).

GEE, L. L., and W. W. SMITH: Defenses against trout furunculosis. J. Bact. 41, 266—267 (1941).

GITLIN, D., and J. M. CRAIG: The thymus and other lymphoid tissues in congenital agammaglobulinemia. I. Thymus alymphoplasia and lymphocytic hypoplasia and their relation to infection. Pediatrics 32, 517—530 (1963).

—, F. S. ROSEN, and C. A. JANEWAY: The thymus and other lymphoid tissues in congenital agammaglobulinemia. II. Delayed hypersensitivity and homograft survival in a child with thymic alymphoplasia. Pediatrics 33, 711—720 (1964).

GLANZMANN, E., und P. RINIKER: Essentielle Lymphocytophthise. Wien. med. Wschr. 100, 35—36 (1950).

GLICK, B., T. S. CHANG, and R. G. JAAP: The bursa of Fabricius and antibody production. Poultry Sci. 35, 224—225 (1956).

— The bursa of Fabricius and the development of immunologic competence. In: The thymus in immunobiology (R. A. GOOD and A. E. GABRIELSEN, eds.). New York: Hoeber-Harper, pp. 343—358.

GLOBERSON, A., and M. FELDMAN: Role of the thymus in restoration of immune reactivity and lymphoid regeneration in irradiated mice. Transplantation 2, 212—227 (1964).

GLOBERSON, A., L. FIORE-DONATI, and M. FELDMAN: On the role of the thymus in recovery of immunological reactivity following X-irradiation. Exp. Cell Res. 28, 455—457 (1962).

GOEDBLOED, J. F., and O. VOS: The capacity for skin rejection in mice thymectomized neonatally or in adult life. Transplantation 3, 368—379 (1965).

GOLDSTEIN, A. L., F. D. SLATER, and A. WHITE: Preparation, assay, and partial purification of a thymic lymphocytopoietic factor (thymosin). Proc. nat. Acad. Sci. (US) 56, 1010—1017 (1966).

Good, R. A., and R. L. Varco: Clinical and experimental study of agamma-globulinemia. J. Lancet 75, 245—271 (1955).

—, A. P. Dalmasso, C. Martinez, O. K. Archer, J. C. Pierce, and B. W. Paper-master: The role of thymus in development of immunologic capacity in rabbits and mice. J. exp. Med. 116, 773—795 (1962).

—, and A. E. Gabrielsen (eds.): The thymus in immunobiology (Conference in Minneapolis, 1962). New York: Hoeber-Harper 1964.

—, and B. W. Papermaster: Ontogeny and phylogeny of adaptive immunity. Adv. Immunol. 4, 1—115 (1964).

—, J. Finstad, B. Pollara, and A. E. Gabrielsen: Morphologic studies on the evolution of the lymphoid tissues among the lower vertebrates. In: Phylogeny of immunity (R. T. Smith, P. A. Miescher, and R. A. Good, eds.). Jacksonville: University of Florida Press 1966, pp. 149—168.

—, M. D. Cooper, R. D. A. Peterson, M. J. Kellum, D. E. R. Sutherland, and A. E. Gabrielsen: The role of the thymus in immune process. Ann. N. Y. Acad. Sci. 135, 451—478 (1966).

— — —, J. R. Hoyer, and A. E. Gabrielsen: Immunological deficiency diseases in man — relationship to disturbances of germinal center formation. In: Germinal centers in immune responses (H. Cottier, N. Odartchenko, R. Schindler, and C. C. Congdon, eds.). Berlin-Heidelberg-New York: Springer 1967, pp. 386—405.

— Discussion remarks. In: Germinal centers in immune responses (H. Cottier, N. Odartchenko, R. Schindler, and C. C. Congdon, eds.). Berlin-Heidelberg-New York: Springer 1967, pp. 209—210 and 457.

Gordon, H. A.: Morphological and physiological characterization of germ free life. Ann. N. Y. Acad. Sci. 78, 208—220 (1959).

Gowans, J. L.: The migration of lymphocytes into lymphoid tissue. In: The thymus in immunobiology (R. A. Good and A. E. Gabrielsen, eds.). New York: Hoeber-Harper 1964, pp. 255—272.

—, and E. J. Knight: The route of recirculation of lymphocytes in the rat. Proc. roy. Soc. Lond. B 159, 257—282 (1964).

Graetzer, M. A., W. P. Cote, and H. R. Wolfe: The effect of bursectomy at different ages on precipitin and natural hemagglutinin production in the chicken. J. Immunol. 91, 576—581 (1963).

Grégoire, C.: Contributions expérimentales à l'étude du thymus des mammifères. Arch. int. Méd. exp. 7, 513—629 (1932).

—, and G. Duchateau: A study on lympho-epithelial symbiosis in thymus. Reactions of the lymphatic tissue to extracts and to implants of epithelial components of thymus. Arch. Biol. Liège 67, 269—296 (1956).

Gross, L.: Effect of thymectomy on development of leukemia in C3H mice inoculated with leukemic "passage" virus. Proc. Soc. exp. Biol. Med. 100, 325—328 (1959).

Hammar, J. A.: Zur Histogenese und Involution der Thymusdrüse. Anat. Anz. 27, 23—30, 41—89 (1905).

— The new views as to the morphology of the thymus gland and their bearing on the problem of the function of the thymus. Endocrinology 5, 543—573, 731—760 (1921).

— Die Lehre vom „Status thymicus" im Lichte der normalen Thymusverhältnisse. Klin. Wschr. 8, 1385—1391 (1929).

— Über die Grundlagen des sog. Status thymicolymphaticus. (Proc. Int. Congr. Pediat., Stockholm, 1930), Acta paediat. 11, 241—256 (1930).

HAMMAR, J. A.: Die normal-morphologische Thymusforschung im letzten Viertel-jahrhundert. Analyse und Synthese nebst einigen Worten zu der Funktionsfrage. Leipzig: Barth 1936.
— Experimentelle Untersuchung über die Rolle der Thymus bei der Immunisierung. Z. mikr.-anat. Forsch. 44, 425—450 (1938).
HAND, T., P. CASTER, and T. D. LUCKEY: Isolation of a thymus hormone, LSH. Biochem. biophys. Res. Comm. 26, 18—23 (1967).
HARBOE, M., H. PANDE, P. BRANDTZAEG, K. J. TVETAR, and P. F. HJORT: Synthesis of donor type γG-globulin following thymus transplantation in hypo-γ-globu-linemia with severe lymphocytopenia. Scand. J. Haemat. 3, 351—374 (1966).
HART, C.: Die Lehre vom Status thymico-lymphaticus. München: Bergmann 1923.
HARRIS, J. E., and C. E. FORD: The role of the thymus, migration of cells from thymic grafts to lymphnodes in mice. Lancet 1, 389—390 (1963).
— — Cellular traffic of the thymus: Experiments with chromosome markers. Evidence that the thymus plays an instructional part. Nature (Lond.) 201, 884 (1964).
HARRIS, T. N., J. RHOADS, and J. STOKES: A study of the role of the thymus and spleen in the formation of antibodies in the rabbit. J. Immunol. 58, 27—32 (1948).
HEINIGER, H. J., H. RIEDWYL, H. GIGER, B. SORDAT, and H. COTTIER: Ultrastruc-tural differences between thymic and lymph node small lymphocytes in mice: nucleolar size and cytoplasmic volume. Blood 30, 288—300 (1967).
HELLMAN, T., und G. WHITE: Das Verhalten des lymphatischen Gewebes während eines Immunisierungsprozesses. Virchows Arch. 278, 221—257 (1930).
HESS, M. W., H. COTTIER, and R. D. STONER: Primary and secondary antitoxin responses in thymectomized mice. J. Immunol. 91, 425—430 (1963).
—, and R. D. STONER: Further studies on antitoxin responses in neonatally thymecto-mized mice. Int. Arch. Allergy 30, 37—47 (1966).
— — Attempts to induce immunological tolerance to tetanus toxoid and xenogeneic lymphoid cells in normal and neonatally thymectomized mice. Path. Microbiol. 30, 155—165 (1967 a).
— — Unpublished results (1967 b).
— —, and H. COTTIER: Growth characteristics of mouse thymus in the neonatal period. Nature (Lond.) 215, 426—428 (1967).
HILDEMANN, W. H.: Scale homotransplantation in the gold fish (Carassius auratus). Ann. N. Y. Acad. Sci. 64, 775—790 (1957).
— Immunogenetic studies of amphibians and reptiles. Ann. N. Y. Acad. Sci. 97, 139—152 (1961).
HILGARD, H. R., K. SJODIN, C. MARTINEZ, and R. A. GOOD: Facilitation of induc-tion of tolerance to allogeneic tissue grafts in adult mice by early thymectomy. Transplantation 2, 638—643 (1964 a).
—, E. J. YUNIS, K. SJODIN, C. MARTINEZ, and R. A. GOOD: Reversal of wasting in thymectomized mice by the injection of syngeneic spleen or thymus cell sus-pensions. Nature (Lond.) 202, 668—670 (1964 b).
HINRICHSEN, K.: Zellteilungen und Zellwanderungen im Thymus der erwachsenen Maus. Z. Zellforsch. 68, 427—444 (1965).
HITZIG, W. H., Z. BIRO, H. BOSCH u. H. J. HUSER: Agammaglobulinaemie und Alymphocytose mit Schwund des lymphatischen Gewebes. Helv. paediat. Acta 13, 551—585 (1958).
—, u. H. WILLI: Hereditäre lympho-plasmocytäre Dysgenesie (Alymphocytose mit Agammaglobulinämie). Schweiz. med. Wschr. 91, 1626—1633 (1961).
—, H. E. M. KAY, and H. COTTIER: Familial lymphopenia with agammaglobulin-aemia. An attempt at treatment by implantation of foetal thymus. Lancet 2, 151—154 (1965).

Holmes, M. C., and F. M. Burnet: Thymic changes in NZB mice and hybrids. In: Thymus. Experimental and clinical studies (G. E. W. Wolstenholme and R. Porter, eds.). London: Churchill 1966, pp. 381—390.

Howie, J. B., and B. J. Helyer: The influence of neonatal thymectomy and thymus grafting on spontaneous autoimmune disease in mice. In: Thymus. Experimental and clinical studies (G. E. W. Wolstenholme and R. Porter, eds.). London: Churchill 1966, pp. 360—380.

Humphrey, J. H., D. M. V. Parrot, and J. East: Studies on globulin and antibody production in mice thymectomized at birth. Immunology 7, 419—439 (1964).

Isakovic, K., B. H. Waksman, and C. Wennersten: Immunologic reactiviy in neonatally thymectomized rats receiving competent lymphoid cells during immunization. J. Immunol. 95, 602—613 (1965 a).

—, S. B. Smith, and B. H. Waksman: Role of the thymus in tolerance. I. Tolerance to bovine gamma globulin in thymectomized, irradiated rats grafted with thymus from tolerant donors. J. exp. Med. 122, 1103—1123 (1965 b).

—, and B. D. Jankovic: Germinal centers and plasma cells in the thymus of the chicken. In: Germinal centers in immune responses (H. Cottier, N. Odartchenko, R. Schindler, and C. C. Congdon, eds.). Berlin-Heidelberg-New York: Springer 1967, pp. 379—382.

Ishidate, M., and D. Metcalf: The pattern of lymphopoiesis in the mouse thymus after cortisone administration or adrenalectomy. Austr. J. exp. Biol. med. Sci. 41, 637—649 (1963).

Janett, A., H. P. Wagner, C. R. Jansen, H. Cottier, and E. P. Cronkite: Studies on lymphopoiesis. IV. A comparison of two approaches for the determination of the generation time in thoracic duct cells without detectable cytoplasmic differentiation. Europ. J. Cancer 2, 231—236 (1966).

Jankovic, B. D., B. H. Waksman, and B. G. Arnason: Role of the thymus in immune reactions in rats. I. The immunologic response to bovine serum albumin (antibody formation, Arthus reactivity and delayed hypersensitivity) in rats thymetomized or splenectomized at various times after birth. J. exp. Med. 116, 159—175 (1962).

Jeejeebhoy, H. F.: Immunological studies on the rat thymectomized in adult life. Immunology 9, 417—425 (1965).

Jerne, N. K., A. A. Nordin, and C. Henry: The agar plaque technique for recognizing antibody-producing cells. In: Cell-bound antibodies (B. Amos and H. Koprowski, eds.). Philadelphia: The Wistar Institute Press 1963, pp. 109—122.

Jeunet, F.: Thymome et syndrome de carence en immunoglobulines. Schweiz. med. Wschr. 95, 1419—1420 (1965).

Joske, R. A.: The effects of thymectomy on the lymphocyte count in patients with myasthenia gravis. Med. J. Aust. 45, 859—861 (1958).

Kadowaki, J. I., W. W. Zuelzer, A. J. Brough, R. I. Thompson, P. V. Woolley, and D. Gruber: XX/XY lymphoid chimaerism in congenital immunological deficiency syndrome with thymic alymphoplasia. Lancet 2, 1152—1156 (1965).

Kalmutz, S. E.: Antibody production in the opossum embryo. Nature (Lond.) 193, 851—853 (1962).

Kalter, S. S., I. A. Ratner, H. A. Britton, T. E. Vice, A. K. Eugster, and A. R. Rodriguez: Wasting syndrome in thymectomized immature baboons (Papio species) after infection with adenovirus type 12. Nature (Lond.) 213, 610—612 (1967).

Kaplan, H. S.: Influence of thymectomy, splenectomy and gonadectomy on incidence of radiation—induced lymphoid tumors in strain C57 black mice. J. nat. Cancer Inst. 11, 83—91 (1950).

Kaplan, H. S.: On the etiology and pathogenesis of the leukemias: A review. Cancer Res. 14, 535—548 (1954).

—, and M. B. Brown: Development of lymphoid tumors in non-irradiated thymic grafts in thymectomized irradiated mice. Science 119, 439—440 (1954).

Kay, H. E. M., J. H. L. Playfair, M. Wolfendale, and P. K. Hopper: Development of the thymus in the human foetus and its relation to immunological potential. Nature (Lond.) 196, 238—240 (1962).

— Personal communication (1967).

Kellum, M. J., and E. Eckert: Morphological and serological abnormalities in rabbits subjected to central lymphoid tissue extirpation and irradiation. Fed. Proc. 24, 491 (1965) (Abstract).

Kemenes, F., and G. Pethes: Further evidence for the role of the bursa of Fabricius in antibody production in chickens. Z. Immun. Forsch. 125, 446—458 (1963).

Kim, Y. B., S. G. Bradley, and D. W. Watson: Ontogeny of the immune response. I. Development of immunoglobulins in germfree and conventional colostrum-deprived piglets. J. Immunol. 97, 52—63 (1966 a).

— — — Ontogeny of the immune response. II. Characterization of 19SγG- and 7SγG-immunoglobulins in the true primary and secondary responses in piglets. J. Immunol. 97, 189—196 (1966 b).

Kindred, J. E.: A quantitative study of the hemopoietic organs of young albino rats. Amer. J. Anat. 67, 99—149 (1940).

— A quantitative study of the hemopoietic organs of adult albino rats. Amer. J. Anat. 71, 207—243 (1942).

Kingsbury, B. F.: The development of the human pharynx. I. The pharyngeal derivatives. Amer. J. Anat. 18, 329—386 (1915).

Klein, J. J., A. L. Goldstein, and A. White: Enhancement of *in vivo* incorporation of labeled precursors into DNA and total protein of mouse lymph nodes after administration of thymic extracts. Proc. nat. Acad. Sci. (Wash.) 53, 812—817 (1965)

— — — Effects of the thymus lymphocytopoietic factor. Ann. N. Y. Acad. Sci. 135, 485—495 (1966).

Klose, H., u. H. Vogt: Klinik und Biologie der Thymusdrüse (mit besonderer Berücksichtigung ihrer Beziehungen zu Knochen- und Nervensystem). Beitr. klin. Chir. 69, 1—200 (1910).

— Chirurgie der Thymusdrüse. Ergebn. Chir. Orthop. 8, 274—423 (1914).

Köbberling, G.: Autoradiographische Untersuchungen über Zellursprung und Zellwanderung in lymphatischen Organen fetaler und neugeborener Mäuse. Z. Zellforsch. 68, 631—659 (1965).

Konda, S., and T. N. Harris: Effect of appendectomy and of thymectomy, with X-irradiation, on the production of antibodies to two protein antigens in young rabbits. J. Immunol. 97, 805—814 (1966).

Kotani, M., K. Seiki, A. Yamashita, and I. Horii: Lymphatic drainage of thymocytes to the circulation in the guinea pig. Blood 27, 511—520 (1966).

Laissue, J., H. Cottier, M. W. Hess, and R. D. Stoner: unpublished observations (1966).

La Via, M. F., D. T. Rowlands, Jr., and M. Block: Antibody formation in embryos. Science 140, 1219—1220 (1963).

Law, L. W., and J. H. Miller: The influence of thymectomy on the incidence of carcinogen-induced leukemia in strain DBA mice. J. nat. Cancer Inst. 11, 425—437 (1950).

—, T. B. Dunn, N. Trainin, and R. H. Levey: Studies of thymic function. In: The thymus (V. Defendi and D. Metcalf, eds.). Philadelphia: The Wistar Institute Press 1964, pp. 105—117.

Law, L. W.: Studies of thymic function with emphasis on the role of the thymus in oncogenesis. Cancer Res. **26**, 551—574 (1966 a).
— Restoration of thymic function in neonatally thymectomized mice bearing xenogeneic thymic grafts. Nature (Lond.) **210**, 1118—1120 (1966 b).
Lazar, A.: Transplantation and function of a histo-incompatible tumour in thymectomized rats. Nature (Lond.) **210**, 1380—1381 (1966).
Leonard, L., and G. McHutchinson: Effect of thymectomy, splenectomy, and irradiation on mouse skin homotransplantation. Transplantation **3**, 343—349 (1965).
Leuchars, E., A. M. Cross, A. J. S. Davies, and V. J. Wallis: A cellular component of thymic function. Nature (Lond.) **203**, 1189—1190 (1964).
— —, and P. Dukor: The restoration of immunological function by thymus grafting in thymectomized irradiated mice. Transplantation **3**, 28—38 (1965).
—, A. J. S. Davies, V. Wallis, and P. C. Koller: Further studies upon mitotic response of thymus derived cells to antigenic stimulation. Ann. N. Y. Acad. Sci. **129**, 274—282 (1966).
Levey, R. H., N. Trainin, L. W. Law, P. H. Black, and W. P. Rowe: Lymphocytic choriomeningitis infection in neonatally thymectomized mice bearing diffusion chambers containing thymus. Science **142**, 483—485 (1963 a).
— — — Evidence for function of thymic tissue in diffusion chambers, implanted in neonatally thymectomized mice. Preliminary report. J. nat. Cancer Inst. **31**, 199—217 (1963 b).
Leyten, R., P. de Somer, P. Denys, Jr., and P. Prinzie: Effect of experimental viral infection in thymectomized rodents. Antonie van Leeuwenhoek J. microbiol. serol. **31**, 145—152 (1965).
Linna, J., and J. Stillström: Migration of cells from the thymus to the spleen in young guinea pigs. Acta path. microbiol. scand. **68**, 465—475 (1966).
Linna, T. J.: Transport of tritium-labelled DNA from the thymus to other lymphoid organs in rabbits under normal conditions and after administration of endotoxin. Int. Arch. Allergy **31**, 313—337 (1967 a).
— Cell migration from the thymus to other lymphoid organs in hamsters of different ages. Uppsala: Student Service 1967 b, pp. 3—38.
Loutit, J. F.: Immunological and trophic functions of lymphocytes. Lancet **2**, 1106—1108 (1962).
Lumb, G. N., and M. O. Symes: On the value of thymectomy in adult mice as a means of potentiating the immunosuppressive action of Melphalan (L-phenylalanine mustard). Immunology **9**, 575—580 (1965).
MacLean, L. D., S. J. Zak, R. L. Varco, and R. A. Good: The role of the thymus in antibody production: An experimental study of the immune response in thymectomized rabbits. Transplant. Bull. **4**, 21—22 (1957).
Marine, D., O. T. Manley, and E. J. Bowman: The influence of thyroidectomy, gonadectomy, suprarenalectomy, and splenectomy on the thymus gland of the rabbit. J. exp. Med. **40**, 429—443 (1924).
Martinez, C., J. Kersey, B. W. Papermaster, and R. A. Good: Skin homograft survival in thymectomized mice. Proc. Soc. exp. Biol. Med. **109**, 193—196 (1962 a).
—, A. Dalmasso, and R. A. Good: Acceptance of tumour homografts by thymectomized mice. Nature (Lond.) **194**, 1289—1290 (1962 b).
—, A. P. Dalmasso, M. Blaese, and R. A. Good: Runt disease produced in thymectomized F_1 hybrid mice injected with parental strain lymphoid cells. Proc. Soc. exp. Biol. Med. **111**, 404—407 (1962 c).
— —, and R. A. Good: Homotransplantation of normal and neoplastic tissue in thymectomized mice. In: The thymus in immunobiology (R. A. Good and A. E. Gabrielsen, eds.). New York: Hoeber-Harper 1964, pp. 465—476.

MATSANIOTIS, N., E. APOSTOLOPOULOU, and J. VLACHOS: Thymic alymphocytosis: Report of a case with normal Peyer's patches. J. Pediat. **69**, 576—582 (1966).

MATSUYAMA, M., M. N. WIADROWSKI, and D. METCALF: Autoradiographic analysis of lymphopoiesis and lymphocyte migration in mice bearing multiple thymic grafts. J. exp. Med. **123**, 559—576 (1966).

MATTI, H.: Untersuchungen über die Wirkung experimenteller Ausschaltung der Thymusdrüse. Ein Beitrag zur Physiologie und Pathologie der Thymus. Mitt. Grenzgeb. Med. Chir. **24**, 665—821 (1911).

MAURER, E. W.: Schilddrüse und Thymus der Teleostier. Morph. Jb. **11**, 129—175 (1886).

MAXIMOW, A.: Untersuchungen über Blut und Bindegewebe. II. Über die Histogenese des Thymus bei Säugetieren. Arch. mikroskop. Anat. **74**, 525—621 (1909).

McINTIRE, K. R., S. SELL, and J. F. A. P. MILLER: Pathogenesis of the post-neonatal thymectomy wasting syndrome. Nature (Lond.) **204**, 151—155 (1964).

McKNEALLY, M., and F. OLIVERAS: Influence of thymectomy in adult dogs. Fed. Proc. **24**, 161 (1965) (Abstract).

MÉTALNIKOV, S. I., et H. GASCHEN: Immunité de la chenille contre divers microbes. C. R. Soc. Biol. **83**, 119—121 (1920).

METCALF, D.: The thymic origin of the plasma lymphocytosis stimulating factor. Brit. J. Cancer **10**, 442—457 (1956).

— The effect of thymectomy on the lymphoid tissues of the mouse. Brit. J. Haemat. **6**, 324—333 (1960).

—, and M. ISHIDATE: PAS-positive reticulum cells in the thymic cortex of high and low leukemia strains of mice. Aust. J. exp. Biol. med. Sci. **40**, 57—71 (1962).

— Functional interactions between the thymus and other organs. In: The thymus (V. DEFENDI and D. METCALF, eds.). Philadelphia: The Wistar Institute Press 1964, pp. 53—72.

— Delayed effect of thymectomy in adult life on immunological competence. Nature (Lond.) **208**, 1336 (1965).

— The thymus. Berlin-Heidelberg-New York: Springer 1966 a.

— The nature and regulation of lymphopoiesis in the normal and neoplastic thymus. In: Thymus. Experimental and clinical studies (G. E. W. WOLSTENHOLME and R. PORTER, eds.). London: Churchill 1966 b, pp. 242—263.

—, and M. BRUMBY: The role of the thymus in the ontogeny of the immune system. J. cell. Physiol. **67** (suppl. 1), 149—168 (1966).

—, and M. WIADROWSKI: Autoradiographic analysis of lymphocyte proliferation in the thymus and in thymic lymphoma tissue. Cancer Res. **26**, 483—489 (1966).

METCHNIKOFF, E.: Immunität bei Infektionskrankheiten. Jena: Fischer 1902.

MEYER, K., M. A. RAO, and R. L. ASPINALL: Inhibition of the development of the bursa of Fabricius in the embryo of the common fowl by 19-nortestosterone. Endocrinology **64**, 890—897 (1959).

MICHALKE, W., H. COTTIER, M. W. HESS, and R. D. STONER: Thymic lymphopoiesis and cell migration in newborn mice: autoradiographic study based on the mitotic labeling pattern after a single injection of ^{3}H-thymidine (1967) (in preparation).

MILLER, J. F. A. P.: Studies on mouse leukaemia. The role of the thymus in leukaemogenesis by cell-free leukaemic filtrates. Brit. J. Cancer **14**, 93—98 (1960).

— Immunological function of the thymus. Lancet **2**, 748—749 (1961).

— Immunological significance of the thymus of the adult mouse. Nature (Lond.) **195**, 1318—1319 (1962 a).

— Role of the thymus in transplantation immunity. Ann. N. Y. Acad. Sci. **99**, 340—354 (1962 b).

MILLER, J. F. A. P.: Tolerance in the thymectomized animal. C. R. Coll. internat. CNRS 116, 47—73 (1963).

—, S. M. A. DOAK, and A. M. CROSS: Role of the thymus in recovery of the immune mechanism in the irradiated adult mouse. Proc. Soc. exp. Biol. Med. 112, 785—792 (1963).

— The thymus and the development of immunologic responsiveness. Science 144, 1544—1551 (1964 a).

— Effect of thymic ablation and replacement. In: The thymus in immunobiology (R. A. GOOD and A. E. GABRIELSEN, eds.). New York: Hoeber-Harper 1964 b, pp. 436—464.

—, and A. J. S. DAVIES: Embryological development of the immune mechanism. Ann. Rev. Med. 15, 23—36 (1964).

—, u. P. DUKOR: Die Biologie des Thymus nach dem heutigen Stande der Forschung. Basel-New York: Karger 1964.

—, and J. G. HOWARD: Some similarities between the neonatal thymectomy syndrome and graft-versus-host disease. J. RES Soc. 1, 369—392 (1964).

—, E. LEUCHARS, A. M. CROSS and P. DUKOR: Immunological role of the thymus in radiation chimeras. Ann. N. Y. Acad. Sci. 120, 205—217 (1964).

— Effect of thymectomy in adult mice on immunological responsiveness. Nature (Lond.) 208, 1337—1338 (1965 a).

— The thymus and transplantation immunity. Brit. med. Bull. 21, 111—117 (1965 b).

—, P. M. DE BURGH, and G. A. GRANT: Thymus and the production of antibody-plaque-forming cells. Nature (Lond.) 208, 1332—1334 (1965).

—, M. BLOCK, D. T. ROWLANDS, JR., and P. KIND: Effect of thymectomy on hemato-poietic organs of the opossum "embryo". Proc. Soc. exp. Biol. Med. 118, 916—921 (1965).

— The thymus in relation to the development of immunological capacity. In: Thymus. Experimental and clinical studies (G. E. W. WOLSTENHOLME and R. PORTER, eds.). London: Churchill 1966, pp. 153—174.

—, P. M. DE BURGH, P. DUKOR, G. GRANT, V. ALLMAN, and W. HOUSE: Regeneration of thymus grafts. II. Effects on immunological capacity. Clin. exp. Immunol. 1, 61—76 (1966).

MITCHELL, A. G. (chairman), E. BOYD, W. E. CHAMBERLAIN, N. H. EINHORN, H. F. HELMHOLZ, and A. H. SPOHN: Panel discussion on the thymus gland. In: Proc. Eighth Ann. Meet. Amer. Acad. Pediat., Del Monte, California; June 9, 1938. J. Pediat. 14, 534—553 (1939).

MORTON, J. I., and B. V. SIEGEL: Hematological changes in mice following Freund's adjuvant administration. Vox Sang. 11, 570—577 (1966).

MUELLER, A. P., H. R. WOLFE, and R. K. MEYER: Precipitin production in chickens. XXI. Antibody production in bursectomized chickens and in chickens injected with 19-nortestosterone on the 5th day of incubation. J. Immunol. 85, 172—179 (1960).

— —, and W. P. COTE: Antibody studies in hormonally and surgically bursectomized chickens. In: The thymus in immunobiology (R. A. GOOD and A. E. GABRIELSEN, eds.). New York: Hoeber-Harper 1964, pp. 359—373.

MURRAY, R. G., and P. A. WOODS: Studies on the fate of lymphocytes. III. The migration and metamorphosis of in situ labeled thymic lymphocytes. Anat. Rec. 150, 113—128 (1964).

NAKAMOTO, O.: The influence of the thymus on the blood picture, especially on lymphocytes. I. Effects of thymectomy on the peripheral blood and lymph nodes. Acta haemat. Jap. 20, 179—187 (1957 a).

NAKAMOTO, O.: The influence of the thymus on the blood picture, especially on lymphocytes. II. Influence of thymic extract on peripheral blood lymphocytes. Acta haemat. Jap. 20, 187—199 (1957 b).

NAKAMURA, K., and D. METCALF: Quantitative cytological studies on thymic lymphoid cells in normal, preleukaemic and leukaemic mice. Brit. J. Cancer 15, 306—315 (1961).

NEZELOF, C., M. L. JAMMET, P. LORTHOLARY, B. LABRUNE et M. LAMY: L'hypoplasie héréditaire du thymus: sa place et sa responsabilité dans une observation d'aplasie lymphocytaire normoplasmacytaire et normoglobulinémique du nourisson. Arch. franç. Pédiat. 21, 897—920 (1964).

NOSSAL, G. J. V.: Studies on the rate of seeding of lymphocytes from the intact guinea pig thymus. Ann. N. Y. Acad. Sci. 120, 171—181 (1964).

—, and J. GORRIE: Studies of the emigration of thymic cells in young guinea pigs. In: The thymus in immunobiology (R. A. GOOD and A. E. GABRIELSEN, eds.). New York: Hoeber-Harper 1964, pp. 288—290.

—, and J. MITCHELL: The thymus in relation to immunological tolerance. In: Thymus. Experimental and clinical studies (G. E. W. WOLSTENHOLME and R. PORTER, eds.). London: Churchill 1966, pp. 105—123.

OKUYAMA, S.: Immunological status of chickens with neonatal thymectomy and bursectomy. II. Serological aspects of thymectomy and bursectomy in chickens. B. Specific antibody production in chickens with neonatal thymectomy and bursectomy. Sci. Rep. Res. Inst. Tohoku Univ., Ser. C 12, 293—296 (1965 a).

— Immunological status of chickens with neonatal thymectomy and bursectomy. III. Delayed hypersensitivity in chickens with neonatal thymectomy and bursectomy. Sci. Rep. Res. Inst. Tohoku Univ., Ser. C 12, 297—302 (1965 b).

OSBORN, J. J., J. DANCIS, and J. F. JULIA: Studies of the immunology of the newborn infant. I. Age and antibody production. Pediatrics 9, 736—744 (1952).

OSOBA, D., and J. F. A. P. MILLER: Evidence for a humoral thymus factor responsible for the maturation of immunological faculty. Nature (Lond.) 199, 653—655 (1963).

— — The lymphoid tissues and immune responses of neonatally thymectomized mice bearing thymus tissue in Millipore diffusion chambers. J. exp. Med. 119, 177—194 (1964).

— The effects of thymus and other lymphoid organs enclosed in Millipore diffusion chambers on neonatally thymectomized mice. J. exp. Med. 122, 633—650 (1965 a).

— Immune reactivity in mice thymectomized soon after birth: normal response after pregnancy. Science 147, 298—299 (1965 b).

— The functions of the thymus. Canad. med. Ass. J. 94, 488—497 (1966).

PAPERMASTER, B. W., R. M. CONDIE, and R. A. GOOD: Immune response in the California hagfish. Nature (Lond.) 196, 355—357 (1962 a).

—, A. P. DALMASSO, C. MARTINEZ, and R. A. GOOD: Suppression of antibody forming capacity with thymectomy in the mouse. Proc. Soc. exp. Biol. Med. 111, 41—43 (1962 b).

—, D. I. FRIEDMAN, and R. A. GOOD: Relationship of the bursa of Fabricius to immunologic responsiveness and homograft immunity in the chicken. Proc. Soc. exp. Biol. Med. 110, 62—64 (1962 c).

PAPPENHEIMER, A. M.: The effects of early extirpations of the thymus in albino rats. J. exp. Med. 19, 319—338 (1914 a).

— Further experiments upon the effects of extirpation of the thymus in rats, with special reference to the alleged production of rachitic lesions. J. exp. Med. 20, 477—498 (1914 b).

Park, E. A., and R. D. McClure: The results of thymus extirpation experiments in the dog. With a review of the experimental literature on thymus extirpation. Amer. J. Dis. Child. 18, 317—354 (1919).

Parrot, D. M. V.: Strain variation in mortality and runt disease in mice thymectomized at birth. Transplant. Bull. 29, 102—104 (1962).

—, and J. East: Role of the thymus in neonatal life. Nature (Lond.) 195, 347—348 (1962).

— — Studies on a fatal wasting syndrome in mice thymectomized at birth. In: The thymus in immunobiology (R. A. Good and A. E. Gabrielsen, eds.). New York: Hoeber-Harper 1964, pp. 523—540.

—, M. A. B. de Sousa, and J. East: Thymus-dependent areas in the lymphoid organs of neonatally thymectomized mice. J. exp. Med. 123, 191—204 (1966).

Paton, D. N., and A. Goodall: Contribution to the physiology of the thymus. J. Physiol. 31, 49—64 (1904).

Perri, G. C., M. Faulk, E. Shapiro, J. Mellors, and W. L. Money: Function of the thymus and growth of tumour homograft. Nature (Lond.) 200, 1294—1296 (1963).

Peterson, R. D. A., W. Kelly, and R. A. Good: Ataxia-telangiectasia, its association with a defective thymus, immunological deficiency disease and malignancy. Lancet 1, 1189—1193 (1964).

Phillips, J. H.: Antibody-like materials of marine invertebrates. Ann. N. Y. Acad. Sci. 90, 760—769 (1960).

Pierce, A. E., R. C. Chubb, and P. L. Long: The significance of the bursa of Fabricius in relation to the synthesis of 7S and 19S immune globulins and specific antibody activity in the fowl. Immunology 10, 321—337 (1966).

Pierpaoli, W., and E. Sorkin: Relationship between thymus and hypophysis. Nature (Lond.) 215, 834—837 (1967).

Pinnas, J. L., and F. W. Fitch: Immunological competence of thymectomized rats to several soluble and particulate antigens. Int. Arch. Allergy 30, 217—230 (1966).

Porter, P. J., A. R. Spievack, and E. H. Kass: The effect of neonatal thymectomy on susceptibility to bacterial endotoxin. J. Lab. clin. Med. 68, 455—462 (1966).

Potter, E. L.: Sudden death in infants. Amer. J. Dis. Child. 76, 435—437 (1948).

Rees, R. J. W.: Enhanced susceptibility of thymectomized and irradiated mice to infection with *Mycobacterium leprae*. Nature (Lond.) 211, 657—658 (1966).

Reinhardt, W. O.: Effect of thymectomy in rats on lymph nodes and spleen. Anat. Rec. 91, 295 (1945) (Abstract).

—, and J. M. Yoffey: Thoracic duct lymph and lymphocytes in the guinea pig. Effects of hypoxia, fasting, evisceration, and treatment with adrenaline. Amer. J. Physiol. 187, 493—500 (1956).

Richer, G., P. Lemonde et A. G. Borduas: Effets de la greffe de thymus homologue et hétérologue chez la souris thymectomisée à la naissance. Rev. canad. Biol. 24, 45—51 (1965).

Roessle, R., u. F. Roulet: Maß und Zahl in der Pathologie. In: Pathologie und Klinik in Einzeldarstellungen. Berlin-Wien: Springer 1932, Band 5.

Rogister, G.: Evolution de la lymphocytose chez la souris "Swiss Albinos". Experientia 20, 266—267 (1964).

— Immunological recovery in neonatally thymectomized "Swiss Albino" mice. Transplantation 3, 669—671 (1965).

Roos, B.: Makrophagensysteme; Hab.-Schrift, Univ. Bern (1967) (in preparation).

Roosa, R. A., D. B. Wilson, and V. Defendi: Effect of thymectomy on hamsters. Proc. Soc. exp. Biol. Med. 118, 584—590 (1965).

Rosen, F. S., D. Gitlin, and C. A. Janeway: Alymphocytosis, agammaglobulinemia, homografts and delayed hypersensitivity: study of a case. Lancet **2**, 380—381 (1962).

—, S. P. Gotoff, J. M. Craig, J. Ritchie, and C. A. Janeway: Further observations on the Swiss type of agammaglobulinemia (alymphocytosis). The effect of syngeneic bone-marrow cells. New Engl. J. Med. **274**, 18—21 (1966).

Rowley, D. A., and F. W. Fitch: The mechanism of tolerance produced in rats to sheep erythrocytes. I. Plaque-forming cell and antibody response to single and multiple injections of antigen. J. exp. Med. **121**, 671—681 (1965 a).

— The mechanism of tolerance produced in rats to sheep erythrocytes. II. The plaque-forming cell and antibody response to multiple injections of antigen begun at birth. J. exp. Med. **121**, 683—695 (1965 b).

Russe, H. P., and A. J. Crowle: A comparison of thymectomized and antithymocyte serum-treated mice in their development of hypersensitivity to protein antigens. J. Immunol. **94**, 74—83 (1965).

Ruth, R. F.: Ontogeny of the blood cells. Fed. Proc. **19**, 579—585 (1960).

Sainte-Marie, G., and C. P. Leblond: Elaboration of a model for the formation of lymphocytes in the thymic cortex of young adult rats. Blood **26**, 765—783 (1965).

Salkind, J.: Contributions histologiques à la biologie comparée du thymus. Arch. Zool. exp. **55**, 81—322 (1915).

Salvin, S. B., R. D. A. Peterson, and R. A. Good: The role of the thymus in resistance to infection and endotoxin toxicity. J. Lab. clin. Med. **65**, 1004—1022 (1965).

Sanders, A. G., and H. W. Florey: The effect of the removal of lymphoid tissue. Brit. J. exp. Path. **21**, 275—287 (1940).

Schaedeli, J., and H. Cottier: Personal communication (1967).

Schinckel, P. G., and K. A. Ferguson: Skin transplantation in the foetal lamb. Austr. J. Biol. Sci. **6**, 533—548 (1953).

Schooley, J. C., and L. S. Kelly: The thymus in lymphocyte production. Fed. Proc. **20**, 71 (1961) (Abstract).

— — Influence of the thymus on the output of thoracic-duct lymphocytes. In: The thymus in immunobiology (R. A. Good and A. E. Gabrielsen, eds.). New York: Hoeber-Harper 1964, pp. 236—253.

— —, E. L. Dobson, C. R. Finney, V. W. Havens, and L. N. Cantor: Reticuloendothelial activity in neonatally thymectomized mice and irradiated mice thymectomized in adult life. J. RES Soc. **2**, 396—405 (1965).

Sherman, J. D., M. M. Adner, and W. Dameshek: Effect of thymectomy on the golden hamster *(Mesocricetus auratus)*. I. Wasting disease. Blood **22**, 252—271 (1963).

— — — Effect of thymectomy on the golden hamster *(Mesocricetus auratus)*. II. Studies of the immune response in thymectomized and splenectomized non-wasted animals. Blood **23**, 375—388 (1964).

Sigel, M. M., and L. W. Clem: Immunological response of an elasmobranch to human influenza virus. Nature (Lond.) **197**, 315—316 (1963).

Silverstein, A. M.: Congenital syphilis and the timing of immunogenesis in the human foetus. Nature (Lond.) **194**, 196—197 (1962).

— Ontogeny of the immune response. Science **144**, 1423—1428 (1964).

—, and K. L. Kraner: Studies on the ontogenesis of the immune response. In: Molecular and cellular basis of antibody formation (J. Sterzl, ed.). Prague-New York-London: Academic Press 1965, pp. 341—348.

—, C. J. Parshall, Jr., and J. W. Uhr: Immunologic maturation *in utero*: Kinetics of the primary antibody response in the fetal lamb. Science **154**, 1675—1677 (1966).

SINCLAIR, N. R.: Haemolysin responses to sheep erythrocytes in neonatally thymectomized Swiss mice. Nature (Lond.) **214**, 95—96 (1967).

SMITH, R. T.: Immunological tolerance of nonliving antigens. Adv. Immunol. **1**, 67—129 (1961).

—, and R. A. BRIDGES: Immunological unresponsiveness in rabbits produced by neonatal injection of defined antigens. J. exp. Med. **108**, 227—250 (1958).

SOLOMON, J. B.: Effects of germ-free environment, bursectomy and irradiation on the production of natural and immune opsonins in young chicks. Immunology **11**, 97—102 (1966).

STANLEY, N. F., H. WARING, and M. YADAV: Discussion remark. In: Thymus. Experimental and clinical studies (G. E. W. WOLSTENHOLME and R. PORTER, eds.). London: Churchill 1966, pp. 207—210.

STARZL, T. E., T. L. MARCHIORO, D. W. TALMAGE, and W. R. WADDELL: Splenectomy and thymectomy in human renal homotransplantation. Proc. Soc. exp. Biol. Med. **113**, 929—932 (1963).

— —, P. I. TERASAKI, K. A. PORTER, T. D. FARIS, T. J. HERRMANN, D. L. VREDEVOE, M. P. HUTT, D. A. OGDEN, and W. R. WADDELL: Chronic survival after human renal homotransplantation. Lymphocyte-antigen matching, pathology and influence of thymectomy. Ann. Surgery **162**, 749—787 (1965).

STERZL, J., and A. M. SILVERSTEIN: Developmental aspects of immunity. Adv. Immunol. **6**, 337—459 (1967).

STÖHR, P.: Über die Abstammung der kleinen Thymusrindenzellen. Anat. Hefte (1. Abt.) **31**, 409—457 (1906).

— Über die Natur der Thymus-Elemente. Anat. Hefte (1. Abt.) **41**, 109—127 (1910).

STOELINGA, G. B. A.: Dysimmunoglobulinaemie bij kinderen. (Med. Diss.) Nijmegen: Centrale Drukkerij 1966.

STRAUSS, A. J. L., and H. W. R. VAN DER GELD: The thymus and human diseases with auto-immune concomitants, with special reference to myasthenia gravis. In: Thymus. Experimental and clinical studies (G. E. W. WOLSTENHOLME and R. PORTER, eds.). London: Churchill 1966, pp. 416—439.

STUTMAN, O., E. J. YUNIS, C. MARTINEZ, and R. A. GOOD: Reversal of post-thymectomy wasting disease in mice by multiple thymus grafts. J. Immunol. **98**, 79—87 (1967).

SUTHERLAND, D. E. R., O. K. ARCHER, and R. A. GOOD: The role of the appendix in development of immunologic capacity. Proc. Soc. exp. Biol. Med. **115**, 673—676 (1964).

—, R. D. A. PETERSON, O. K. ARCHER, E. ECKERT, and R. A. GOOD: Development of "autoimmune processes" in rabbits after neonatal removal of central lymphoid tissue. Lancet **1**, 130—133 (1965).

SVET-MOLDAVSKY, G. J., S. N. ZINZAR, and N. M. SPECTOR: Dissociation of the immunological competence in neonatally thymectomized mice and its restoration. Nature (Lond.) **202**, 353—355 (1964).

SZENBERG, A., and N. L. WARNER: Dissociation of immunological responsiveness in fowls with a hormonally arrested development of lymphoid tissue. Nature (Lond.) **194**, 146 (1962 a).

— — Quantitative aspects of the Simonsen phenomenon. I. The role of the large lymphocyte. Brit. J. exp. Path. **43**, 123—128 (1962 b).

SZENT-GYORGYI, A., A. HEGYELI, and J. A. McLAUGHLIN: Cancer therapy: A possible new approach. Science **140**, 1391—1392 (1963).

TAITZ, L. S., C. ZARATE-SALVADOR, and E. SCHWARTZ: Congenital absence of the parathyroid and thymus glands in an infant (III and IV Pharyngeal Pouch Syndrome). Pediatrics **38**, 412—418 (1966).

TAKEYA, K., R. MORI, and K. NOMOTO: Antibody-forming cells of neonatally thymectomized mice. Proc. Jap. Acad. 40, 572—575 (1964).

—, and K. NOMOTO: Development of immunological capacities in normal and thymectomized mice. Nature (Lond.) 213, 1248—1249 (1967).

TAYLOR, R. B.: Decay of immunological responsiveness after thymectomy in adult life. Nature (Lond.) 208, 1334—1335 (1965).

TESSERAUX, H.: Physiologie und Pathologie des Thymus, unter besonderer Berücksichtigung der pathologischen Morphologie. Leipzig: Barth 1953.

THIEFFRY, S., M. ARTHUIS, J. AICARDI et G. LYON: L'ataxie-téléangiectasie. Rev. neurol. 105, 390—405 (1961).

THOMAS, E.: Klinik und Pathologie des Status thymico-lymphaticus. Jena: Fischer 1927.

THORBECKE, G. J., H. A. GORDON, B. S. WOSTMANN, M. WAGNER, and J. A. REYNIERS: Lymphoid tissue and serum gamma globulin in young germfree chickens. J. infect. Dis. 101, 237—251 (1957).

TING, R. C., and L. W. LAW: The role of thymus in transplantation resistance induced by polyoma virus. J. nat. Cancer Inst. 34, 521—527 (1965).

TOBLER, R., und H. COTTIER: Familiäre Lymphopenie mit Agammaglobulinämie und schwerer Monoliasis. Helv. paediat. Acta 13, 313—338 (1958).

TOULLET, F. T., and B. H. WAKSMAN: Role of the thymus in tolerance. IV. Specific tolerance to homografts in neonatally thymectomized mice grafted with thymus from tolerant donors. J. Immunol. 97, 686—692 (1966).

TRAININ, N., L. W. LAW, and R. H. LEVEY: Patterns of reconstitution of neonatally thymectomized mice by injection of isolated lymphopoietic and hemopoietic cells. Proc. Soc. exp. Biol. Med. 118, 79—85 (1965).

—, A. BEJERANO, M. STRAHILEVITCH, D. GOLDRING, and M. SMALL: A thymic factor preventing wasting and influencing lymphopoiesis in mice. Israel J. med. Sci. 2, 549—559 (1966).

TRENCH, C. A. H., J. W. WATSON, F. C. WALKER, P. S. GARDNER, and C. A. GREEN: Evidence for a humoral thymic factor in rabbits. Immunology 10, 187—191 (1966).

TYAN, M. L., and L. J. COLE: An impairment of antibody production in adoptively restored, lethally irradiated thymectomized mice. Clin. exp. Immunol. 2, 121—131 (1967).

VAN FURTH, R., H. R. E. SCHUIT, and W. HIJMANS: The immunological development of the human fetus. J. exp. Med. 122, 1173—1188 (1965).

WAKSMAN, B. H., B. G. ARNASON, and B. D. JANKOVIC: Role of the thymus in immune reactions in rats. III. Changes in the lymphoid organs of thymectomized rats. J. exp. Med. 116, 187—205 (1962).

WARNER, N. L., A. SZENBERG, and F. M. BURNET: The immunological role of different lymphoid organs in the chicken. I. Dissociation of immunological responsiveness. Aust. J. exp. biol. med. Sci. 40, 373—387 (1962).

— — Immunological reactivity of bursaless chickens in graft versus host reactions. Nature (Lond.) 199, 43—44 (1963).

— — Immunologic studies on hormonally bursectomized and surgically thymectomized chickens: Dissociation of immunologic responsiveness. In: The thymus in immunobiology (R. A. GOOD and A. E. GABRIELSEN, eds.). New York: Hoeber-Harper 1964, pp. 395—411.

WEISSMAN, I. L.: Thymus cell migration. J. exp. Med. 126, 291—304 (1967).

WILSON, R., K. SJODIN, and M. BEALMEAR: Thymus studies in germfree (axenic) mice. In: The thymus (V. DEFENDI and D. METCALF, eds.). Philadelphia: The Wistar Institute Press 1964 a, pp. 89—93.

Wilson, R., K. Sjopin, and M. Bealmear: The absence of wasting in thymectomized
    germfree (axenic) mice. Proc. Soc. exp. Biol. Med. **117**, 237—239 (1964 b).
Wilson, R. J. M., V. E. Jones, and S. Leskowitz: Thymectomy and anaphylactic
    antibody in rats infected with *Nippostrongylus brasiliensis*. Nature (Lond.) **213**,
    398—399 (1967).
Wolstenholme, G. E. W., and R. Porter (eds.): The thymus: Experimental and
    clinical studies. (CIBA Symposium.) London: Churchill 1966.
Wong, F. M., R. N. Taub, J. D. Sherman, and W. Dameshek: Effect of thymus en-
    closed in Millipore diffusion envelopes on thymectomized hamsters. Blood **28**,
    40—53 (1966).
Yunis, E. J., C. Martinez, J. Smith, and R. A. Good: Facilitation of host lymphoid
    tissue development in neonatally thymectomized mice by injection of allogeneic
    dispersed thymus cells. Nature (Lond.) **204**, 750—853 (1964).
—, H. R. Hilgard, C. Martinez, and R. A. Good: Studies on immunologic recon-
    stitution of thymectomized mice. J. exp. Med. **121**, 607—632 (1965).
Zinzar, S. N., and G. J. Svet-Moldavsky: Features of antibody formation in neo-
    natally thymectomized mice. Nature (Lond.) **214**, 295—297 (1967).

Subject Index

Herstellung: Konrad Triltsch, Graphischer Betrieb, Würzburg

Experimentelle Medizin, Pathologie und Klinik

Die früheren Bände erschienen unter dem Reihentitel:

Pathologie und Klinik in Einzeldarstellungen